Nursing Leadership From
the Outside In

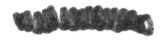

Greer Glazer, PhD, RN, CNP, FAAN, is Dean, College of Nursing, Schmidlapp Professor of Nursing, University of Cincinnati, Cincinnati, Ohio. A distinguished scholar and an international leader in nursing education, service, and research, Dr. Glazer has 30 years of experience in the field of women's health. She holds a PhD and MSN in nursing from Case Western Reserve University and a BSN from the University of Michigan. Previously, she was Dean and Professor, College of Nursing and Health Sciences, University of Massachusetts Boston, and Professor and Director of Parent Child Nursing, Kent State's College of Nursing. Dr. Glazer completed a 3-year Robert Wood Johnson Executive Nurse Fellowship from 2001 to 2004. She was a Fulbright Scholar at Tel Aviv University, Israel, in 2004 and provided consultation to the Israeli Ministry of Health. She has done extensive research on women's health, including the institutionalization of domestic violence education and support programs in health care institutions and barriers to the provision and utilization of prenatal health care services for African American women. As chairperson of the Political Action Committee of the American Nurses Association, she oversaw fund-raising activities. Dr. Glazer is widely published, is in great demand as a public speaker, and has appeared on numerous radio and television programs. She is a cofounder and current Legislative Editor of the *Online Journal of Issues in Nursing*.

Joyce J. Fitzpatrick, PhD, MBA, RN, FAAN, is the Elizabeth Brooks Ford Professor of Nursing, Frances Payne Bolton School of Nursing, Case Western Reserve University, Cleveland, Ohio, where she was Dean from 1982 through 1997. She edits three journals: *Nursing Education Perspectives,* the flagship journal of the National League for Nursing, *Applied Nursing Research*, and *Archives of Psychiatric Nursing*. Dr. Fitzpatrick has received numerous honors and awards, including the *American Journal of Nursing* Book of the Year Award 18 times. Dr. Fitzpatrick is widely published in nursing and health care literature. She is former Senior Editor for the *Annual Review of Nursing Research* and a well-published Springer Publishing Company author and editor. She founded and led the Bolton School's World Health Organization Collaborating Center for Nursing. She has provided consultation on nursing education and research throughout the world, including universities and health ministries in Africa, Asia, Australia, Europe, Latin America, and the Middle East. She served as a Fulbright Scholar at University College Cork in Ireland. She currently serves as Chair of the American Nurses Foundation Board of Trustees.

Nursing Leadership From the Outside In

Greer Glazer, PhD, RN, CNP, FAAN
Joyce J. Fitzpatrick, PhD, MBA, RN, FAAN
Editors

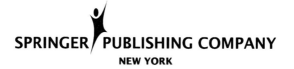

SPRINGER PUBLISHING COMPANY
NEW YORK

Springer Publishing Company, LLC
11 West 42nd Street
New York, NY 10036
www.springerpub.com

Acquisitions Editor: Allan Graubard
Production Editor: Michael O'Connor
Composition: S4Carlisle Publishing Services

ISBN: 978-0-8261-0866-1
e-book ISBN: 978-0-8261-0867-8

13 14 15 16 / 5 4 3 2

The author and the publisher of this Work have made every effort to use sources believed to be reliable to provide information that is accurate and compatible with the standards generally accepted at the time of publication. Because medical science is continually advancing, our knowledge base continues to expand. Therefore, as new information becomes available, changes in procedures become necessary. We recommend that the reader always consult current research and specific institutional policies before performing any clinical procedure. The author and publisher shall not be liable for any special, consequential, or exemplary damages resulting, in whole or in part, from the readers' use of, or reliance on, the information contained in this book. The publisher has no responsibility for the persistence or accuracy of URLs for external or third-party Internet websites referred to in this publication and does not guarantee that any content on such websites is, or will remain, accurate or appropriate.

Library of Congress Cataloging-in-Publication Data
Nursing leadership from the outside in / Greer Glazer, Joyce J. Fitzpatrick, editors.
    p. ; cm.
Includes bibliographical references and index.
ISBN 978-0-8261-0866-1 — ISBN 0-8261-0866-0 — ISBN 978-0-8261-0867-8 (e-book)
I. Glazer, Greer Lita. II. Fitzpatrick, Joyce J., 1944-
[DNLM: 1. Leadership. 2. Nursing—organization & administration. 3. Professional
Competence. WY 105]
610.73068—dc23   2012044486

Printed in the United States of America by Gasch Printing.

Contents

Contributors

Martin Alpert, MD
Founder and Former President
   of Cumulus Corporation
Founder and Former Chairman
   and President of Tecmar, Inc.
Solon, Ohio

Amy V. Blue, PhD
Assistant Provost for
   Education
Medical University of South
   Carolina
Charleston, South Carolina

Carol A. Cartwright, PhD
President (retired)
Kent State University
   (1991–2006)
Bowling Green State
   University (2008–2011)
Bowling Green, Ohio

Michael F. Collins, MD
Chancellor
University of Massachusetts
   Medical School
Worcester, Massachusetts

Arthur G. Cosby, PhD
William L. Giles Distinguished
   Professor and Director
Social Science Research Center
Mississippi State University
Starkville, Mississippi

Jerry Cromwell, PhD
Economist, Senior Fellow in
   Health Economics
Research Triangle Institute
Waltham, Massachusetts

Michael J. Dowling
Chief Executive Officer
North Shore-LIJ Health
   System
Great Neck, New York

Victor J. Dzau, MD
Chancellor for Health Affairs
   and James B. Duke Professor
   of Medicine
Duke University
President, Duke University
   Health System
Durham, North Carolina

**Joyce J. Fitzpatrick, PhD,
   MBA, RN, FAAN**
Elizabeth Brooks Ford
   Professor of Nursing
Frances Payne Bolton School
   of Nursing
Case Western Reserve
   University
Cleveland, Ohio

Catherine L. Gilliss, PhD, RN, FAAN
Dean and Helene Fuld Health
  Trust Professor of Nursing
Duke University School of
  Nursing
Vice Chancellor for Nursing
  Affairs, Duke University
Durham, North Carolina

Greer Glazer, PhD, RN, CNP, FAAN
Dean, College of Nursing
Schmidlapp Professor of
  Nursing
University of Cincinnati
Cincinnati, Ohio

Karen Gross, JD
President
Southern Vermont College
Bennington, Vermont

Wylecia Wiggs Harris, PhD, CAE
Chief of Staff
American Nurses Association
Silver Spring, Maryland

Kate Judge
Executive Director
American Nurses Foundation
Silver Spring, Maryland

Steven C. LaTourette
U.S. House of Representatives,
  Ohio, 14th District, 1994–2013
Washington, DC

Johnnie Maier
Former State Representative
Ohio House of Representatives
Massillon Municipal Clerk of
  Court
Massillon, Ohio

Shawn D. Mathis, MA
Chairman, Board of Directors
The Onsomblé Inc. (formerly
  The Nurse Company, Inc.)
Nashville, Tennessee

Joan Mazzolini, MA
Communications Officer
Sisters of Charity Foundation
Cleveland, Ohio

David C. Pate, MD, JD, FACP, FACHE
President and Chief Executive
  Officer
St. Luke's Health System
Boise, Idaho

Al Patterson, PharmD
Director of Pharmacy
Boston Children's Hospital
Boston, Massachusetts

Scott Reistad, RRT, CPFT, FAARC
Director Respiratory Care,
  Sleep Labs, and Caring
  Excellence
St. Anthony Hospital
Lakewood, Colorado

Anne Rosewarne
President
Michigan Health Council
Okemos, Michigan

Barry H. Smith, MD, PhD
President
Dreyfus Health Foundation
New York, New York

Derek van Amerongen, MD, MS
Chief Medical Officer
Humana of Ohio
Cincinnati, Ohio

Steven A. Wartman, MD, PhD, MACP
President and Chief Executive Officer
Association of Academic Health Centers
Washington, DC

Louise Woerner, MBA, FAAN
Executive Board Chair
HCR Home Care
Rochester, New York

Foreword

*N*ursing Leadership From the Outside In by Greer Glazer and Joyce J. Fitzpatrick offers leadership lessons for aspiring nurse leaders from luminaries in business, medicine, philanthropy, government, academia, research, and health care. These nurse champions know firsthand the potential for nurses to help transform health care and improve patient care, as well as the myriad obstacles we face in making our voices heard. As businessman Shawn D. Mathis states in his chapter, "The true leaders of the health care industry are on the front lines of health care delivery."

But nurses know all too well that we are seldom at the policy and decision-making tables to influence the debate on how to improve health care. A recent survey of 1,000 hospitals in the United States by the American Hospital Association (AHA) found that nurses account for only 6% of hospital board members. In comparison, physicians account for 20% of board members, and other clinicians make up about 5% of hospital board members (AHA, 2011).

Nevertheless, health care leaders desire nurses to have more influence. A recent Gallup poll of 1,500 health opinion leaders said they wanted nurses to have more influence in a variety of areas, especially in reducing medical errors, increasing quality of care, and promoting wellness. They also believed that nurses should have more input and impact in planning, policy development, and management (Robert Wood Johnson Foundation, 2010).

The Robert Wood Johnson Foundation (RWJF) strongly believes that nurses, as the largest segment of the health care workforce and the providers who spend the most time with patients, must be central to efforts to improve health care. That is why we have invested over $300 million in nursing programs in the past 10 years and why we support numerous nursing leadership programs, including our flagship *RWJF Executive Nurse Fellows* program, in which Greer Glazer participated from 2001 to 2004. I am proud that Greer Glazer is coediting this book with Joyce J. Fitzpatrick.

She continues our storied tradition of our alumni working to improve the health and health care of all Americans.

RWJF's nationwide Future of Nursing: Campaign for Action, which we lead along with AARP seeks to ensure that all Americans have access to high-quality, patient-centered health care by advancing the recommendations of the Institute of Medicine report, *The Future of Nursing: Leading Change, Advancing Health.* A major focus of the Campaign is to work at the national and state levels to transform our health care system by ensuring that nurses are part of management discussions and health care policy debates. Nurses must be at the table when decisions are being made about patient care delivery.

This book, if adopted widely, will prepare and enable nurses to lead change to advance health. *Nursing Leadership From the Outside In* offers practical advice, lessons learned, and testimonials as to how nurses can prepare themselves for leadership, which in turn, will help them to provide exceptional patient care.

Schools of nursing, leadership programs, and nursing associations throughout the United States should make this book required reading. Readers should heed the words of the American Nurses Association's Wylecia Wiggs Harris, chief of staff and special projects officer: "take from this book what is relevant to help you grow and become a transformational leader well positioned to participate in and lead collaborative dialogue in advancing health care."

It is my hope that nurses at all stages of their careers and at all levels will follow the advice of the health care leaders in *Nursing Leadership From the Outside In*. As Greer Glazer notes in her Introduction, there has "never been a better time to prepare nurse leaders to transform health care." Take the lessons here, apply them, and become the leaders we so desperately need to improve health and health care for all Americans. With *The Future of Nursing: Leading Change, Advancing Health* serving as the blueprint to transform the nursing field and improve patient care and its offering of detailed advice, all nurses will be able to help make history by implementing important strategies to ensure great patient care for all.

Susan B. Hassmiller, PhD, RN, FAAN
Senior Advisor for Nursing
Robert Wood Johnson Foundation
Silver Spring, Maryland

REFERENCES

American Hospital Association (AHA). (2011). *AHA Hospital Statistics, 2010 edition*. Chicago, IL: Author.

Committee on the Robert Wood Johnson Foundation Initiative on the Future of Nursing at the Institute of Medicine. (2010). *The future of nursing: Leading change, advancing health*. Washington, DC: National Academies Press.

RWJF. (2010). Nursing Leadership from Bedside to Boardroom. Retrieved from http://www.rwjf.org/en/research-publications/find-rwjf-research/2010/01/nursing-leadership-from-bedside-to-boardroom.html

Publisher's Perspective

When Joyce Fitzpatrick and Greer Glazer first approached me with their idea to publish a book on nursing leadership *from the outside in*, I was immediately attracted. Here was a pertinent, vivacious perspective that involved interprofessional collaboration on many levels, from the macro to the micro. It was also a perspective that nurse leaders knew well by virtue of their experience in education, and in the practice, policy, and industry arenas. When have nurse leaders not worked with other health science leaders, government officials, political appointees, and private industry captains on diverse issues that inform and structure health science, its economics, and the way care and cure are provided? At the same time, I had not yet seen a book dedicated to this collaboration with this particular point of view. Although nursing leadership books mention or discuss interprofessional collaboration, it is more than rare to find content about nurse leaders and the leadership they provide from leaders in other fields.

There is a kind of insular quality within nursing, and the discourse about nurse leadership, that this book avoids. Certainly, this grows more important with the recent Institute of Medicine document that calls for nursing to collaborate openly and horizontally, and at all levels, with its health science colleagues. Stating the need, however, does not clarify or resolve the distinctions among disciplines, nor does it offer a means to do so, especially in terms of power relationships and the kind of authority rooted in those relationships.

How can health science, the health care industry, and health policy make best use of its largest professional workforce and how can that workforce make best use of them? In another sense, how can nurse leaders best use their positions within a practice environment that is currently more integrated than the academic environment, and, I must add, within both as a continuum of learning and doing?

This book, although certainly not a first step in responding to these questions, does open up, or more broadly open, a dimension that nurse leaders face on a daily basis: how they are viewed by those who work with them. It is both a reflection and a refraction of what nurse leaders offer, what they have offered, and what they will offer in a society in which health care largely remains a commodity for purchase by individuals. In the United States, we have yet to achieve what other countries have achieved and profit by: universal health care coverage.

Understanding how others view you is important in recognizing how best to work with them. That truism is no less true for being a truism. It is what this book takes to heart. I also hope it is a sign that publishers will respond with speed and discretion to new conditions, needs, hopes, and strategies that now inform and seek to reform nursing leadership, from the ground up.

Allan Graubard
Former Executive Editor
Springer Publishing

Acknowledgments

I have stood on the shoulders of giants in nursing. My early and subsequent exposure to exemplary nursing leaders including Jan Bellack, Becky Bergman, Gaurdia Bannister, Shirley Chater, Marilyn Chow, Joyce Clifford, Rosemary Ellis, Jeanette Ives Erickson, Jacqueline Fawcett, Vernice Ferguson, Joyce J. Fitzpatrick, Nancy Lytle, Pat Reid Ponte, Rozella Schlotfeldt, and May Wykle, have fueled my passions for nursing and assuring that nurses are at the table to provide our unique contribution to the health of people and communities. My brother, Gary Glazer, and father, Norman Glazer, national physician leaders, provided me with an early interdisciplinary perspective and mentored me in leadership from the beginning of my career. All of my efforts would not have been possible without the tremendous support of my family who have endured a commuter marriage for 8½ years—my husband, Kerry Volsky, and children Jessica, Hannah, and Norman Volsky. Thank you to Angela Clark, a PhD student at the University of Cincinnati, who assisted with all aspects of this book. Thank you also to the contributing authors with expertise in government, medicine, academia, nursing, health care management, and leadership for sharing their life experiences.

Greer Glazer

I echo the words of my colleague, Greer Glazer. Those of us in leadership positions today have learned from the trailblazing work of our predecessors. Without leaders and mentors in nursing and health care the nursing profession would not be as advanced as it is today. I also add my thanks to the chapter contributors. Current and future nurse leaders will benefit greatly from your insights and advice. I would like to acknowledge the work of the doctoral students from Case Western Reserve University Frances Payne Bolton School of Nursing, Margaret Delaney, Margaret Murphy, Mary Beth Modic, and Erin Ross, who identified key focus areas for the chapters and provided editing insights in their earliest versions. Thank you.

Joyce J. Fitzpatrick

1

Introduction

Greer Glazer

Since the beginning of civilization the groundwork and expectations for nursing practice have been in a state of constant transformation in response to the personal, community, and global health needs of the times. The increasingly more complex, diverse, and interdisciplinary facets of the health care system prompted the Institute of Medicine and the Robert Wood Johnson Foundation to join together and assess the current state of health care, thus issuing a "call to action" by the nursing profession. This monumental report challenges nurses to practice to the full extent of their training, achieve higher levels of education, transform health care and improve research and information systems. The heightened roles of the professional nurse allow nurses of all practices to more fully develop their leadership skills. Throughout my career I have closely observed the intraprofessional workings of nurse leaders and borrowed lessons from leaders of other fields to enhance my practice. *Nursing Leadership From the Outside In* showcases perspectives on nursing from a dynamic composite of successful leaders and offers guidance and insight while motivating and empowering even the most accomplished professional.

My personal and professional life changed in April 2001 when I was notified by the Robert Wood Johnson Executive Nurse Fellows (RWJENF) Program that I was a finalist for their leadership program. I was invited to New York for an interview that would determine the awardees. The interviewers asked me a question that was identical to a question on the written application, and I felt well prepared to answer. The question was, "Who do you want to be your mentor during this program?" I confidently replied that I felt that the dean of the top-ranked school of nursing would be an outstanding mentor. Without missing a beat, the interviewer replied that as an experienced nurse executive, I certainly had spent enough time with nurse leaders. One goal of

1

the RWJENF program was to expose nurses to excellent leaders in other disciplines. There was a wealth of information that non-nurses could teach nurses about how they viewed nursing, health care, and leadership that would expand my worldview, network, and potential to influence and transform health care. This was a revelation to me as I believe it was to the other Fellows who were selected. It was time to stop talking to ourselves and to listen to and learn from the expertise of others. I ended up being mentored by then Congressman and current Senator Sherrod Brown and Dr. Lois Nora, former dean of the Northeastern Ohio University College of Medicine. I learned very much about leadership from these nonnurses: one a politician and the other a physician. The importance of knowing people from other disciplines and professions, understanding their perspectives, learning from them, and jointly working together toward common goals (that would be different if you considered only one point of view) was a lesson that I learned for which I am grateful. The idea to edit a book on how others perceive nursing leadership was a natural evolution of my RWJENF experience.

There has never been a better time to prepare nurse leaders to transform health care. The Robert Wood Johnson Foundation (RWJF) approached the Institute of Medicine (IOM) in 2008 to propose a partnership to assess and respond to the need to transform the nursing profession. They believed that this initiative for the future of nursing, coupled with health care reform resulting from the signing into law of Patient Protection of the Health Care Affordability Act on March 10, 2010, created a unique opportunity to transform the health care system. The transformation would result in improved health outcomes by increasing access and quality, promoting wellness and disease prevention, reducing health disparities, providing compassionate care across the lifespan, and slowing health care costs.

An 18-member interdisciplinary committee was appointed that included six nurses. They had five meetings, three public forums, searched the literature, collected testimony, held site visits, commissioned research papers, and sought public input to gather information (IOM, 2011). Their report, *The Future of Nursing: Leading Change, Advancing Health* (2011), was published and disseminated widely on November 30, 2010. The significance of the IOM releasing this report is that the National Academy of Sciences is charged to provide unbiased and authoritative advice to decision makers and the public to improve health. In addition, this was not a report written by nurses about nurses. This is the first national report on nursing with recommendations that are evidence based. One would think that most nurses would be familiar with the IOM report and its recommendations. In my conversations with practicing nurses; students in baccalaureate, master's, Doctor of Nursing Practice (DNP), and PhD programs; and educators throughout the country, I have been amazed that most are unaware of this landmark report, and if they do know about the report, cannot cite more than a few of the recommendations. *The Future of Nursing: Leading Change, Advancing Health* has four key messages and eight recommendations that will serve as a blueprint for charting the future of nursing. Key messages are as follows:

1. Nurses should be able to practice to the full extent of their education and training.
2. Nurses should achieve higher levels of education and training through an improved education system that promotes seamless academic progression.
3. Nurses should be full partners with physicians and others in redesigning U.S. health care.
4. Effective workforce planning and policy making require better data collection and an information infrastructure (IOM, 2011, p. 4).

The eight recommendations are as follows:

1. Remove scope-of-practice barriers (p. 9).
2. Expand opportunities for nurses to *lead* and diffuse collaborative improvement efforts (p. 11).
3. Implement nurse residency programs (p. 11).
4. Increase the proportion of nurses with BSN degrees to 80% by 2020 (p. 12).
5. Double the number of nurses with a doctorate by 2020 (p. 13).
6. Ensure that nurses engage in lifelong learning (p. 13).
7. Prepare and enable nurses to *lead* change to advance health (p. 14).
8. Build an infrastructure to collect and analyze health care workforce data (p. 14).

Two of the eight recommendations specifically use the word "lead," and the others indirectly relate to the need for nursing leadership. A flashback to my RWJENF experience reminds me that it is not enough to make sure that all nurses know about the IOM report. If nurses are going to lead the transformation of health care, we need physicians, politicians, insurance executives, health care chief executive officers, consumers, everyone, to join our efforts.

Leadership has been a competency of the RWJENF program; an American Association of Colleges of Nursing (AACN) BSN, MSN, and DNP essential; a National League of Nursing (NLN) baccalaureate, master's and doctoral program competency; a "Health Professionals for a New Century" transformative learning objective (Frenk et al., 2010); and among the Interprofessional Education Collaborative Expert Panel's *Core Competencies for Interprofessional Collaborative Practice* (2011).

The RWJENF Program was developed by Ed O'Neil and Associates at the University of California, San Francisco in 1997 to "inspire senior level nurses in executive roles to continue the journey toward achieving the highest levels of leadership in the health care system of the 21st century" (RWJF, 2008b). The five core competencies of the program were self-knowledge and self-renewal; inspiring and leading change; risk taking and creativity; strategic vision; and interpersonal and communication effectiveness (RWJF, 2008a). The RWJENF program office transitioned to the Center for Creative Leadership (CCL) at the University of North Carolina Chapel Hill in 2011.

The retooled RWJENF Program goal is to "create a cadre of nursing leaders with enhanced leadership capacity who drive improvements in population health; access, cost, and quality of American Health Systems, and the identification and formation of future health professionals" (CCL, 2011, slide 3). The four major competencies are *leading self* (increasing self-awareness, developing adaptability, managing yourself, learning agility, and leading with purpose); *leading others* (managing effective teams and workgroups, building and maintaining relationships, leveraging diversity and difference, developing others, and communicating effectively); *leading the organization* (leading change, solving problems, making decisions and managing work, managing politics and influencing others, boundary spanning, and setting vision and strategy), and *leading health care* (exerting leadership in and through professional organizations, exerting leadership on boards and expert panels, exerting leadership in interprofessional contexts, exerting leadership through political/legislative action, and exerting leadership by improving health care) (RWJF, 2012).

AACN, which represents baccalaureate and higher degree programs, has developed essential competencies for baccalaureate, master's, and DNP programs that include leadership.

Baccalaureate essential II is "Basic Organizational and Systems Leadership for Quality Care and Patient Safety" (AACN, 2008). The baccalaureate nurse is expected to practice in complex health care systems and assume the role of provider of care; designer/manager/coordinator of care; and member of the nursing profession. The master's-prepared nurse is expected to manage complex systems of care by exhibiting flexible leadership and critical action (AACN, 2011). Master's prepared nurses are leaders in all settings in which health care is delivered. They assume roles of clinician, outcomes manager, advocate, educator, systems analyst/risk anticipator, and leader and partner in the interprofessional health care team. Master's essential II, "Organizational and System Leadership," builds on the baccalaureate competency to prepare master's nurses for management roles at the microsystem level by initiating and maintaining effective interprofessional working relationships using respectful communication, collaborations, care coordination, delegation, and initiating conflict-resolution strategies. They assume a leadership role in effectively implementing patient safety and quality improvement initiatives (AACN, 2011).

DNP programs are designed to prepare nurses for the highest level of leadership in practice that is innovative, evidence based, and reflects application of research. DNP graduates assume roles of APN (nurse practitioners, clinical nurse specialists, nurse anesthetists, and nurse midwives), organizational leadership/administrative roles, and policy roles. DNP essential II, "Organizational and Systems Leadership for Quality Improvement and Systems Thinking," builds on the baccalaureate and master's competencies by adding the ability to conceptualize feasible new care delivery models based on nursing science and organizational, political, cultural, and economic realities. DNP graduates assume accountability for the quality of health care and patient safety for panels of patients, a target population, set of population health systems or community using principles of business, finance, economics, and health policy (AACN, 2006).

NLN, the voice for nursing education that includes associate degree and diploma nursing programs, embeds leadership in the professional-identity competency for baccalaureate, master's and doctoral programs. A baccalaureate nurse will express one's identity as a nurse by exhibiting a "willingness" to provide leadership in "improving care" (NLN, 2011). Master's-prepared nurses will implement one's advanced practice role by demonstrating leadership, promoting positive change in people and systems, and advancing the profession. Competencies for graduates of practice doctorates do not include the word "leadership"; however, leadership competencies are necessary in order to attain NLN DNP competencies in designing and implementing changes in nursing practice and health policy that will serve a diverse population and diverse nursing workforce.

The International Council of Nurses (ICN) has been a pioneer in leadership development for nurses for over 25 years. ICN identified Leadership for Change (LFC) as one of three key program areas (pillars) crucial to the betterment of nursing and health, and its activities are focused in these areas. ICN recognized that leadership is essential for nurses to be involved in health internationally.

> Those who are or will be in key leadership and management positions need to be adequately prepared to help shape policy, work effectively in interdisciplinary teams, plan and manage effective and cost-efficient services, involve communities and key stakeholders in health care planning and delivery, and prepare other nurse managers and leaders for the future. (ICN, 2011a)

ICN developed the LFC program to change the current situation in which

> nurses are often perceived as traditional and reactive, and not as leaders who could have an important contribution to broader health service policy development and management. Nurses' potential or confidence to operate in many ways is often not clear to themselves. (ICN, 2011a)

ICN's program is based on the premise that nurses need to be prepared for leadership not only in nursing but also in health service. The ICN also has a Global Nursing Leadership Institute, "an advanced leadership program for nurses and/or midwives in senior level and executive positions." This program enables senior/executive nurses to "enhance their national and global leadership knowledge and skills" (ICN, 2011c). Participants in this program are expected to be able to form strategic national and global alliances, understand health care globally, and assume leadership positions nationally and globally. The Leadership in Negotiation program is the other thrust of ICN's leadership development strategy (ICN, 2011b).

Leadership competencies are being recognized as essential to other health professions as well as nursing. The Interprofessional Education Collaborative (sponsored by the AACN, American Association of Osteopathic Medicine, American Association of Colleges of Pharmacy, American Dental Education Association, Association of American Medical Colleges, and Association of Schools of Public Health) identified core competencies for interprofessional collaborative practice. Their vision is that interprofessional collaborative practice is critical to safe, quality, accessible patient-centered care. Specific team and teamwork competencies include "apply leadership practices that support collaborative practice and team effectiveness." Graduates of nursing (and other health profession) programs are expected to demonstrate leadership in advancing effective interprofessional collaboration through reflection, promotion of effective decision making, identification of barriers to collaboration, flexibility and adaptability, ability to assume different roles on teams and be supportive of others on teams, and establish and maintain effective working relationships with individuals, families, and organizations to achieve common goals (Interprofessional Education Collaborative Expert Panel, 2011).

The Commission on Education of Health Professionals for the 21st century was formed in January 2010 to develop recommendations that would transform education in nursing, medicine, and public health with the goal of strengthening health systems in an interdependent world. This Commission included 20 people representing diverse disciplines and countries. The report, "Health Professionals for a New Century: Transforming Education to Strengthen Health Systems in an Interdependent World," was published in *The Lancet* (www.thelancet.com, DOI:10.1016/S0140-6736(10)61854-5). The vision of this group is that

> all health professionals in all countries should be educated to mobilize knowledge and to engage in critical reasoning and ethical conduct so that they are competent to participate in patient and population-centered health systems as members of locally responsive and globally connected teams. The ultimate purpose is to assure universal coverage of the high quality comprehensive services that are essential to advance opportunity for health equity within and between countries. (Frenk et al., 2010, p. 3)

In order to realize this vision, transformative learning and interdependence in education will be required. Transformative learning is about developing leadership attributes for the purpose of producing enlightened change agents (Frenk et al., 2010).

There are consistent key messages contained in all of the documents and programs previously described. First, leadership is an essential competency for all nurses. Another example of this key message is the work of the American Nurses Association (ANA). In 2011, ANA introduced a program to profile all nurses as leaders, sponsoring a YouTube video contest for nurses. The winning video, submitted by a school nurse, was very powerful, profiling her leadership qualities in every aspect of her everyday work.

As the educational level increases, leadership competencies move from patient centered to groups of patients, communities, and systems. Second, nurses must develop leadership competencies that enable them to lead beyond nursing to all of health care. The transformation of health care will require interprofessional education and practice. Last, the community has expanded from local practice to a global environment. Leadership competencies are needed that enable nurses to become members of globally connected teams. Leadership competency is identified as a key competency for all nursing (and other health professions) practice; however, leadership is rarely defined.

DEFINITIONS OF LEADERSHIP

Here lies a man who attracted better people into his service
than he was himself.
— ANDREW CARNEGIE

Leadership and management are not the same thing; however, many people use these terms interchangeably and researchers often confuse these concepts. Leadership theories from 1900 to 1970 centered on personal traits of leaders (great leaders are born that way), behaviors and skills (great leaders do these things), and organizational context (doing the right thing at the right time). None of these theories resulted in definitive or practically useful knowledge about leadership (Sashkin & Sashkin, 2003). James McGregor Burns, a historian, wrote in 1978 that "leadership is one of the most observed and least understood phenomena on earth" (Burns, 1978, p. 2). He developed a new paradigm of leadership called transformational leadership that contrasted with the previous theories that were characterized as transactional leadership. In transformational leadership, leaders transform followers into more capable self-directed leaders. On the basis of Kohlberg's (1973) theory, Burns summarizes that "transforming leadership ultimately becomes moral in that it raises the level of human conduct and ethical aspirations of both leader and led, and thus it has a transforming effect on both" (Burns, 1978, p. 20). Many leadership experts distinguish transactional and transformational leaders by noting that transactional leaders base relationships with followers on a process of "barter," whereas transformational leaders base the relationship on bonding (Sergiovanni, 2000). Sashkin and Sashkin (2003) synthesized the work of leadership scholars to identify eight key elements of leadership: communication, trust, caring, creating opportunities, self-confidence, empowerment of others, vision, and organizational content. Transformational leaders include members of organizations working together as partners to construct a new organizational culture that motivates, changes, and empowers people and organizations for the better. Effective leaders are caring, self-confident people who have and effectively communicate a vision to followers who plan together how to make the vision a reality by developing trust and empowering others and by creating opportunities for change for the best throughout an organization. Burns defines leadership as

> leaders inducing followers to act for certain goals that represent the values and motivations—the wants and needs, the aspirations and expectations—of both leaders and followers. . . . Leadership over human beings is exercised when persons with certain motives and purposes mobilize, in competition or conflict with others, institutional, political, psychological, and other resources so as to arouse, engage, and satisfy the motives of followers. (Burns, 1978, p. 18)

Tichy and Devanna (1986) identified seven attributes of transformational leaders. They (1) trust their own intuitions; (2) believe in people and attend to their needs; (3) identify and articulate their own core values; (4) are not afraid to take risks; (5) see themselves as change agents; (6) are flexible and open to new ideas; and (7) are disciplined, careful thinkers. Drucker (1995), the father of modern management, "knew" four "simple" things about effective leaders: (1) the only definition of a leader is someone who has followers; (2) an effective leader is not someone who is loved or admired. He or she is someone whose followers do the right thing; (3) leaders are highly visible and set examples; and (4) leadership is not titles, rank, privileges, or money. It is responsibility. Although leadership and management are related, they are not the same concept. Zaleznik (1981) wrote a classic article on the difference between managers and leaders, arguing that they differ in their personal characteristics and history; motivation; how they think and act; and their orientation toward goals, work relationships, and worldviews. Differences between leadership and management (Grossman & Valiga, 2009) are exaggerated for the purpose of illustration in Table 1.1.

A major point is that leadership is not necessarily linked to a position of authority. Using Burns's definition of leadership, that leaders transform followers into leaders, each of us has the ability to provide leadership whoever we are. We have the potential, and responsibility, to provide leadership in our practice, organizations, community, and the world. Leadership can be learned.

> Strong leadership is likely the single most important driver of overall organizational performance. . . . Nowhere is the need for effective leadership more pronounced than in the

TABLE 1.1
Differences Between Leadership and Management

	Leadership	Management
Position	Selected or allowed by a group of followers	Appointed by someone higher in the organizational hierarchy
Power base	Comes from knowledge, credibility, and ability to motivate followers	Arises from one's position of authority
Goals/visions	Arises from personal interests and passion that may not be synonymous with the goals of the organization	Espoused or prescribed by the organization
Innovative ideas	Developed, tested, and encouraged among all members of the group	Allowed, provided they do not interfere with task accomplishment, but not necessarily encouraged
Risk level	High risk, creativity, innovation	Low risk, balance, maintaining the status quo
Degree of order	Relative disorder seems to be generated	Rationality and control prevail
Nature of activities	Related to vision and judgment	Related to efficiency and cost-effectiveness
Focus	People	Systems and structure
Perspective	Long range, with an eye on the horizon	Short range, with an eye on the bottom line
Degree of "freedom"	Freestanding and not limited to an organizational position of authority	Tied to a designated position in an organization
Actions	Does the right thing (Bennis & Nanus, 1985, p. 21)	Does things right (Bennis & Nanus, 1985, p. 21)

dynamic, complex health care industry, where leaders face unprecedented pressure to transform their organizations so as to meet growing demands for high quality and effective care. In fact, to meet the ambitious expectations of health reform (to reduce cost and simultaneously assure high quality) and to meet the goals laid out by the Institute of Medicine—that is to develop a safe, effective, patient-centered, timely, efficient, and equitable system—the industry needs to better prepare men and women to manage the complex organizations that provide and finance care. (National Center for Healthcare Leadership, 2010, p. 1)

The IOM Report; health care reform; and new educational competencies for baccalaureate, master's, and doctoral students have provided nurses with the opportunity of a lifetime to lead the transformation of health care. Our leadership will be dependent on others' perceptions of our ability to lead, their acceptance of being followers and team members, and our skill and ability to lead. It is our hope that having nonnurses share their thoughts about leadership and experiences with nurse leaders will help us take off our blinders. We can learn by example and apply the knowledge to become better leaders. The time for nurses to lead is now.

REFERENCES

American Association of Colleges of Nursing. (2006). *The essentials of doctoral education for advanced nursing practice.* Retrieved April 17, 2012, from www.aacn.nche.edu/publications/position/dnpessentials.pdf

American Association of Colleges of Nursing. (2008). *The essentials of baccalaureate education for professional nursing practice.* Retrieved April 17, 2012, from www.aacn.nche.edu/education-resources/BaccEssentials 08.pdf

American Association of Colleges of Nursing. (2011). *The essentials of master's education in nursing.* Retrieved April 17, 2012, from www.aacn .nche.edu/educationresources/MastersEssentials11.pdf

Bennis, W., & Nanus, B. (1985). *Leaders: The strategies for taking charge.* New York: Harper & Row.

Burns, J. M. (1978). *Leadership.* New York, NY: Harper & Row.

Center for Creative Leadership. (2011). *Robert Wood Johnson Foundation Executive Nurse Fellows informational applicant web conference, November 7, 2011* [PowerPoint slides]. Retrieved from http://www.executive nursefellows.org/

Drucker, P. (1995). *Managing in a time of great change.* New York, NY: Truman Talley Books/Dutton.

Frenk, J., Chen, L., Bhutta, Z. A., Cohen, J., Crisp, N., Evans, T., . . . Zurayk, H. (2010, November). Health professionals for a new century: Transforming education to strengthen health systems in an interdependent world. *The Lancet, 376*, 1923–1958.

Grossman, S. C., & Valiga, T. M. (2009). *The new leadership challenge: Creating the future of nursing* (3rd ed.). Philadelphia, PA: F.A. Davis.

Institute of Medicine. (2011). *The future of nursing: Leading change, advancing health*. Washington, DC: The National Academies Press.

International Council of Nurses. (2011a). Background [Leadership for Change program]. Retrieved from http://www.icn.ch/pillarsprograms/background/

International Council of Nurses. (2011b). The leadership in negotiation. Retrieved from http://www.icn.ch/pillarsprograms/leadership-in-negotiation/

International Council of Nurses. (2011c). What is the ICN Global Nursing Leadership Institute? Retrieved from http://www.icn.ch/pillarsprograms/what-is-the-icn-global-nursing-leadership-institute/

Interprofessional Education Collaborative Expert Panel. (2011). *Core competencies for interprofessional collaborative practice: Report of an expert panel*. Washington, DC: Interprofessional Education Collaborative.

Kohlberg, L. (1973). The claim to moral adequacy of a highest stage of moral judgment. *Journal of Philosophy, 70*(18), 630–646. doi:10.2307/2025030. JSTOR 2025030.

National Center for Healthcare Leadership. (2010). *Best practices in health leadership talent management and succession planning: Case studies*. Retrieved April 18, 2012, from www.nchl.org/Documents/Ctrl.../doccopy5306_uid72120111204372.pdf

National League of Nursing. (2011). Competencies for graduates of baccalaureate programs. Retrieved from http://www.nln.org/facultydevelopment/Competencies/comp_bacc.htm

Robert Wood Johnson Foundation. (2008a). *Executive Nurse Fellows 2007–2008 call for applications* [PDF document]. Retrieved from www.rwjf.org/files/applications/cfp/cfp_execnurse0708.pdf

Robert Wood Johnson Foundation. (2008b). Retrieved from http://www.rwjf.org/content/dam/files/legacy-files/article-files/2/rwjf scholarsfellows.pdf

Robert Wood Johnson Foundation. (2011). *Robert Wood Johnson Foundation Executive Nurse Fellows program results report*. Retrieved from http://www.rwjf.org/pr/product.jsp?id=17968

Robert Wood Johnson Foundation. (2012). *Robert Wood Johnson Foundation Executive Nurse Fellows*. Retrieved from http://www.rwjfleaders.org/programs/robert-wood-johnson-foundation-executive-nurse-fellows-program

Sashkin, M., & Sashkin, M. G. (2003). *Leadership that matters*. San Francisco, CA: Berrett-Koehler.

Sergiovanni, T. J. (2000). *The lifeworld of leadership*. San Francisco, CA: Jossey Bass.

Tichy, N. M., & Devanna, M. A. (1986). *The transformational leader*. New York, NY: John Wiley.

Zaleznik, A. (1981). Managers and leaders: Are they different? *Journal of Nursing Administration, 11*(7), 25–31. (Originally published by *Harvard Business Review*, May–June 1977.)

2

Nursing: A New Paradigm

Martin Alpert

Commentary
by Joyce J. Fitzpatrick

*A*lpert *is a businessman, and he suggests a new business for nurses. He challenges nurses to capture the market for least invasive therapies, which he labels least invasive therapies and evaluations (LITE), that can be used and are being used by many individuals for a range of symptoms and health conditions. He describes this innovative leadership approach as a way for nurses to be independent, have fun, earn more money, and most important, improve patient care.*

Many of the therapies that Alpert suggests are already being used by individuals as supplements to their traditional medical care. Often, the patients do not inform their providers about their use of complementary and alternative therapies. Thus, the least invasive therapies that Alpert suggests may not be monitored or evaluated. This is the area suggested for nursing. No doubt it would require a paradigm shift for many nurse leaders whose work is embedded within the traditional care delivery system.

Alpert challenges all of us to think of new modalities for health care delivery, highlighting the fact that the current system is unsustainable, both in terms of the high cost and the often deleterious outcomes of traditional interventions. Nurse leaders should consider leading in the area of LITE and heed Alpert's call to action in a new model of health care. As more nurses

> *assume key roles in primary care, it will be possible to integrate these least invasive therapies into the health promotion and symptom management components of care that are so much a part of nursing's understandings of their contribution to health care. If nurses do not take the lead in this new approach, there will be other practitioners who fill the void.*

Key focus areas: independent, courage, opportunity, leadership of nursing, entrepreneur, check your ego

> *The doctor of the future will give no medicine, but will interest his patients in the care of the human frame, in diet, and in the cause and prevention of disease*
> — THOMAS ALVA EDISON

My intent here is not to praise nursing, but to challenge nursing. In my experience, there is plenty of praise for nursing and some blame, but neither of these will be addressed here. I am not going to discuss leadership in nursing, but leadership of nursing. I present a method by which individual nurses can be independent, improve patient care, have fun, and earn more money. More than that, you will have opportunities to achieve better patient outcomes and, occasionally, these better results cannot be attained any other way. You will help more people by practicing under the fundamental principle of medicine: *Do no harm.*

Currently, medicine is in disarray. We use the latest, most aggressive, and high-tech therapies, which are usually the most expensive, instead of the least invasive, least toxic, and least expensive therapies. The current situation is not sustainable. I propose that the nursing profession become the leader in a shift to sustainable, least invasive therapies and evaluations (LITE). These therapies are also usually the least expensive. LITE represents a major profit opportunity for nurses. Many of these new therapies require medical professionals, but not necessarily doctors. They can be administered by dedicated and trained nurses. This strategy will significantly reduce society's medical expenses while potentially *improving* patient medical outcomes. My primary focus is on what is currently referred to as complementary or alternative medicine (CAM), or integrative medical techniques, but not exclusively. Know your profession: when, where, and for how long to use LITE and when to stop using it or when not to use it at all and use conventional therapy. You will need to use your judgment, and good medical judgment means knowing your limits.

As many medical specialties have evolved, they acquire new clinical responsibilities. For example, pulmonary medicine has become the leader in sleep and allergy medicine. Hematology does oncology. I propose that nurses become leaders and "specialists" in LITE. Nurses can become LITE specialists. Although my intent is that this new nursing specialty encompass a wide variety of therapies, I will focus on a subset of what could be available to nursing as leaders in "least invasive" medicine. I am not proposing that each nurse become a specialist in all of them, but that nursing, as a profession, encompass all of them.

The impact of LITE on the global society of nursing leading this area of medicine could be transformational for nursing, medicine, and society. My own interest is in applying these techniques in developing countries. In the same way, some developing countries have leapfrogged the West in going directly to cellular as the primary communication system, seldom using landlines; these same countries could leapfrog and promote the use of advanced noninvasive therapies and achieve better results than the West.

I will mention a few more techniques briefly. Acupuncture is becoming part of conventional therapy. It can be a part of nursing practice. I experienced relief from tennis elbow with acupuncture, administered by an incredibly competent nurse. She also treated me to reduce swelling for a torn Achilles tendon before surgery. I also had acupuncture after surgery. The physical therapists commented that they had never seen anyone heal this fast, which is not the way I typically heal.

The main point I want to convey is that nurses, as medical professionals, should not be followers, but leaders in an area that could pioneer one of the most important changes in medicine in history. Nursing could lead in diagnosis and treatment under the LITE paradigm. I am suggesting that nursing spearhead this approach. The current path of medicine destroys many lives. It also helps many lives, but the costs will eventually destroy society. The Six-Million Dollar Man is not jumping over buildings, but is in the intensive care unit for 6 months.

It will require a lot of courage for nursing to take this on. The "medical establishment" has a lot to lose. It affects their control, money, and power. The stakes are high, professionally and monetarily. The money spent on complementary medicine now exceeds out-of-pocket money spent on conventional medicine.

"Herbal" medicine—also called botanical medicine or phytomedicine—refers to using a plant's seeds, berries, roots, leaves, bark, or flowers for medicinal purposes. Herbalism has a long tradition of use outside of conventional medicine. It is becoming more mainstream as improvements in analysis and quality control, along with advances in clinical research, show the value of herbal medicine in treating and preventing disease.

Recently, the World Health Organization estimated that 80% of people worldwide rely on herbal medicines for some part of their primary health care. On a trip to Rwanda, our guide in the rainforest said there were about 1,100 different species in the rainforest and 80% of them had medicinal value. In the last 20 years in the United States, public dissatisfaction with the cost of prescription medications, combined with an interest in returning to natural or organic remedies, has led to an increase in herbal medicine use. Many factors determine how effective a herb will be. For example, the type of environment (climate, bugs, soil quality) in which a plant grew will affect it, as will how and when it was harvested and processed. Herbal medicine is used to treat many conditions, such as asthma, eczema, premenstrual syndrome, rheumatoid arthritis, migraine, menopausal symptoms, chronic fatigue, and irritable bowel syndrome.

I hope I have convinced you that there is an opportunity here for nurses and nursing. Now I would like to investigate how to implement this approach and what leadership would be required to implement this new paradigm. First, I recommend that nursing schools develop a department of LITE. This will legitimize the practice of these techniques and define nursing as the leader, researcher, and main practitioners of these techniques. Nursing schools could provide courses in different LITE specialties leading to certification in these specialties along with a nursing degree. Occasionally, certification may require an additional year, or even 2 years of education.

Nursing schools should not refer to these as CAM. They are not. It is my intent to make these least invasive techniques the first line of medical care wherever they are applicable. More invasive techniques are appropriate when these fail or are not applicable. In other words, conventional medicine becomes complementary. This will decrease the pressure on current medical staff and decrease medical costs. Funding for research, education, and implementing LITE will probably have to come from the private sector. I do not believe the current medical infrastructure will support this new approach.

Individual nurses may choose to start their own practice or business. This is the area in which I have personally experienced my greatest successes (and failures). Starting your own business is a lot of fun, especially when successful, but it can be scary; I would stress not to be afraid. I need to warn you, though, that my own experience contradicts almost everything taught by formal business courses. In fact, I did my best in business until I learned business, and then things deteriorated. A business person starts with what he or she has and sees how far it can go; an entrepreneur starts with a goal and sees how to get there. You will need to be entrepreneurs. If you have a good basic strategy, you can make many mistakes and still be very successful. I made so many repeated mistakes, I actually learned from some of them. Hiring the right people is critical and is the area I failed the most in. I express this as a caution; the people you work with may determine whether the business succeeds or fails. I have a few additional comments. Check your ego. As success builds, so does the ego, and I have seen many companies go under owing to the founder's ego. Finally, the company takes on the characteristics of its head. If you do not like what you see in your company, take a good look inside yourself.

There is a new trend in business in which business is between bits, not people. This will continue, but business between people will become more common, as it was in the past; especially in the type of business that you will start. You will interact directly with people, so your reputation, both personally and professionally, will be very important.

Wealth is created by business. Your business will participate in this because the next major area of social change, I believe, will come from biological sciences. During my parents' generation, their lives were changed by mechanics, cars, and planes, and the icon representing this was Henry Ford. In my generation, it was computers and communications, and the icon is Bill Gates. But for the next generation, it will be biological sciences. I predict that for the generation that follows them, it will be the arts (unless we really mess things up, which is likely), where personal growth will be most important.

Finally, I want to take this opportunity to make some recommendations for nursing that are not directly related to what I have written here. It affects end-of-life patients, primarily those in hospice. The first is easy: play music that these patients like; maintain their appearance, comb their hair, cut their nails, and so on. It makes the transition more pleasant and dignified. Second, I think each person should have the option to leave a statement or enter the following information into a website describing the life lessons they learned, what was important to them, what they want to pass on to others, and so forth. Some of the questions to ask are:

1. What would you have done differently?
2. What was most important in your life retrospectively?
3. What do you want to be remembered for?
4. What do you want to apologize for (which could be published posthumously or during life)?
5. What lessons would you like to pass on to the next generation?
6. Would you like to describe your life?
7. What are you happy about in regard to what you have done or have?
8. What would you like others to do after you are gone?
9. How has your attitude changed as you got older?
10. What do you recommend to the younger generation?
11. Do you feel good about your life?
    a. Why or why not?
    b. If you do, what makes you feel good about your life?
    c. If not, what would you do to feel good about your life?

These questions might make the person's life more meaningful and death less painful.

Nurses should also consider asking similar, though modified, questions to all their patients. It could give their patients a new way of thinking while they are being treated and also give them more reasons and motivation to get well.

In the end, it is not what you have, but what you do that counts, so I would like to leave you with one last thought,

"What do **you** want to be remembered for?"

3

Nursing Leadership in an Era of Collaboration

Amy V. Blue

Commentary
by Joyce J. Fitzpatrick

*B*lue's recommendations for collaboration are *especially timely given the 2010 Robert Wood Johnson (RWJ) report on the* Future of Nursing *(2010). Interprofessional education and collaboration among health professionals are embedded in the RWJ recommendations, and many universities are implementing changes to address collaboration in the educational process in the expectation of effecting change at the service delivery level. Leadership can occur at many levels. As the Provost at a university with a health science focus, Blue is familiar with the need for participatory change within the curricula of the health science schools.*

Blue's advice to nurse leaders is to apply their creative pragmatism to problem solving, avoid strident positions, use the skills that are basic to nursing, that is, interpersonal and communication skills, and be certain to follow through with expected activities and fulfill responsibilities. Accordingly, nurse leaders should disavow themselves of the perception of inferiority and avoid working from the shared mentality of an historically disempowered profession vis-à-vis medicine. The focus on interpersonal

> *and communication skills is especially important for nurse leaders to nurture in future leaders. Although in nursing we consistently acknowledge the value of interpersonal relationships, we also often forget that these skills apply as much to our boardroom interactions as to our work at the bedside.*

Key focus areas: action, vision, collaboration, pragmatism, communication

The provision of health care is a complex enterprise and spans a multitude of domains, such as individual patient care, community health, health care delivery systems, and health professions education and training. Interprofessional education (IPE) and collaborative practice are increasingly called upon to improve these domains' respective and overlapping spheres of activity with the larger goal of improving the overall health care system. Effective leadership within this era of increased interprofessional collaboration is critical for the success of developing a collaborative practice-ready workforce, and for the creation and sustainability of collaborative health systems. Nurse leaders are moving the interprofessional collaboration agenda forward by serving in key leadership positions nationally and on local campuses. Through application of effective leadership skills and role-modeling behavior, they are fostering a culture shift within our health care system and its associated educational programs.

It is through this work in IPE that I have interacted with a variety of nurse leaders in and beyond my university. Currently, I am the assistant provost for education at the Medical University of South Carolina (MUSC), Charleston, South Carolina, with primary responsibilities of developing and implementing the institution's IPE initiative across the campus. MUSC is an academic health center composed of six colleges: dental, graduate studies, health professions, medicine, nursing, and pharmacy. Our college of nursing offers the only accelerated BSN degree nursing program in South Carolina, as well as DNP, PhD, and MSN programs of study. The college is a leader in online nursing education. Prior to my appointment in the provost's office, I was the associate dean for curriculum and evaluation in the MUSC college of medicine and had been involved exclusively in medical education for nearly 15 years. My educational background as a medical/health professions educator is a little unusual because my doctorate is in medical anthropology. Following a 2-year National Institute of Mental Health postdoctoral fellowship at the University of Kentucky (UK) College of Medicine in the Department of Behavioral Science, my career shifted to medical education through continued work at UK with the college's medical curriculum revision in the early 1990s. Through mentoring and collaboration with outstanding medical educators at both UK and MUSC, I developed my knowledge and skills in medical education. During the last few years, I have transferred my medical education expertise to health professions education and work with students and faculty across the health professions on our campus and through national IPE activities. As a nonphysician, moving out of a physician-centered world to the broader realm of health professions education has been enlightening and instructive and has afforded me the opportunity to interact with leaders from multiple professions with differing styles of leadership.

Definitions of leadership are many. A year ago, I presented about leadership to our pharmacy students, and to reference the plethora of literature on this topic, I found over 365,371 book titles about leadership listed on Amazon.com. Leadership has been studied in multiple ways. Some have examined it as action, with an associated set of behaviors and skills. Others have focused on leadership as a trait, with particular characteristics. And still other researchers have examined it as a relationship. My ideas of leadership stem from the literature and personal experience, including my interactions with leaders and my own leadership attempts.

Leadership occurs at multiple levels and varies by context. Commonly we think about leadership, particularly in academic health care, as the university president, the college dean, or department chair. But leadership occurs within the context of committees, classrooms, clinical environments, and so on. The nuanced layers of what constitutes leadership struck me once during an event for students when the staff and students present did not know what to do and the designated leader was inept at bringing any direction to the situation. A colleague murmured to me, "We need some leadership here." Her statement inferred that action was needed at the time to provide direction to the group. Thus in my definition, an important element of leadership is taking action when needed and providing direction. For me, a great leader is creative, respectful and compassionate, accountable, collaborative, and genuinely listens to, and accommodates, different perspectives in a situation. Finally, leadership should be about improving the greater good and looking to serve the interests of others. It should not be used to advance one's own ambitions.

In reflecting on leadership lessons for nurse leaders, I draw upon multiple interactions with nurses at my institution and during work with national committees. A disclaimer is needed: My comments and examples are not meant to offend or ungraciously stereotype. Nursing, as is true of all professions, attracts a wide range of personalities and talents. Although the examples I provide are based upon interactions with nursing colleagues, I recognize that knowledge, behaviors, personal characteristics, and attitudes are not entirely unique to a particular profession. Illustrated examples I reference could be based upon persons represented in other professions. However, in keeping with the assignment, I have focused on illustrations based upon my work with nurses. Finally, for purposes of organizing this chapter, I thought of several emerging nurse leaders I know and framed my thoughts around recommendations I would share with them. This is not meant to be an exhaustive set of recommendations, nor to reflect on each aspect of leadership I previously defined. Rather, the list was developed in tandem with reflection on positive and negative interactions with nurse leaders and effective leadership behaviors and characteristics.

RECOGNIZE YOUR UNIQUE PROFESSIONAL COMPETENCIES AND SHARE THEM WITH PASSION

Leaders are individuals, who not only possess leadership skills, but typically also possess competency in their profession; they excel in their discipline. They also possess a vision and passion to share that vision with others. Nurse leaders, through a combination of their training, professional experiences, and personal preferences, have unique knowledge and skills for which they are enthusiastic champions. Although all health professionals have a common goal of ensuring optimal health for patients and communities, nurses possess unique training and a professional model for health prevention, promotion, and patient care. This professional perspective is not always explicitly known to other health professionals. The astute nurse leader recognizes the unique contributions she or he can make and, in turn, shares them passionately with others.

A few examples come to mind to illustrate this recommendation. Several of our nursing faculty members at MUSC are experts in community-based participatory research and community health. Applying their enthusiasm for this work, they provide mentoring to other nonnursing faculty and students interested in community health efforts. In one of our IPE programs for students, the Presidential Scholars Program, our nursing faculty members are always strong advocates for students' project work to link with the community in a meaningful and sustainable fashion. Through facilitation with students in the Scholars Program, these Scholars nursing faculty members teach and role model successful strategies for working with the community to improve community health. They also demonstrate for the other nonnursing Scholars faculty these important skills. By sharing their knowledge and skills of effective community-based work and partnerships, as well as their passion for it, our nursing faculty members demonstrate effective leadership in this key area for our campus.

Another illustration of nurses providing leadership through sharing their passion based upon unique knowledge and skills is the increased attention to social determinants of health in our MUSC academic programs' curricula. A few years ago, the Center for Community Health Partnerships in the College of Nursing at MUSC hosted a series of town hall meetings to present the *Unnatural Causes* documentary series about social determinants of health (SDOH). The goal was to inform and engage the campus in a common activity focused on improving the community's health. Through attendance at these presentations, faculty, staff, and students across campus became better informed about SDOH, several of us learning about this concept for the first time. Faculties in other academic programs were excited to learn about SDOH and the video series, recognizing the concept as a powerful explanatory model and the video series as an engaging instructional tool. A mini-revolution was sparked with faculty members incorporating learning objectives associated with SDOH into academic programs to better inform our students about how social factors impact the health of individuals and communities. By sharing their passion for and their unique knowledge of SDOH, our nurse leaders on campus improved the learning environment for both faculty and students.

AVOID A STRIDENT STANCE

At times, enthusiasm and vision for a concept or action plan can generate within the leader such a passion that it appears that other perspectives are not heard, appreciated, or valued; a bigger picture may be lost through a singular, clamorous focus. Avoid this tendency, one I refer to as a "strident stance" and that others may conceptualize as "pushy." I am unsure whether this characteristic stems from an underlying lack of confidence that others will not grasp and value the vision, or whether it emanates from what some term a traditional self-perception of "nurse oppression" in health care. Whatever the source, it is ultimately not helpful and will turn others away from the message being delivered. Insistence upon the value of one's opinion is important. However, I have occasionally observed nurse leaders neglect to recognize others' thoughts, perspectives, and contributions on an issue and forge ahead with a plan. Those individuals who perceived their opinions ignored or shut out became more passive in the group effort and their contributions lost. In some situations, the insistence upon a singular point by a nurse leader becomes framed by other individuals as the only issue of interest held by the nurse leader to the unnecessary exclusion of other associated and important issues. Effective nurse leaders frame their messages through words and actions intent on galvanizing broad input and diverse opinion to achieve a better solution (see section on working collaboratively).

APPLY YOUR CREATIVE PRAGMATISM
TO PROBLEM SOLVING

Leaders are creative and willing to take risks. They are also looked upon for solving problems and problem solving that is realistic. Leaders lose credibility if proposed solutions appear impractical and unrealistic. I find many nurse leaders are creative and pragmatic individuals who skillfully combine these characteristics to address problems and determine effective solutions. To illustrate this ability, I draw upon my experience working with an interprofessional faculty group to develop our first required interprofessional course on campus. As a group, we were discussing possible ways to deliver such a course with the challenge of students' different daily schedules; it appeared that most academic programs have their students in class the majority of the day, and we recognized programs would be resistant to giving us substantive time for class meetings. Our nurse colleague suggested an online approach, educating the group about her experience with online teaching in the college. For several members of the group, online learning represented an innovative approach because other academic programs on campus have incorporated little online learning in their programs. The practical benefits of this delivery method to work around the issue of class timetables were recognized by all of us. The group proceeded to develop the course as a primarily online experience for students. Our nursing colleague provided important leadership for our efforts through offering a creative and pragmatic solution to an issue, allowing us as a group to collectively move forward toward our goal.

In a different professional situation, a nurse leader offered a practical and, in the context, creative solution to resolve a sensitive authorship issue. In a group writing effort of a manuscript, one lead author felt particular individuals should be included as coauthors and another lead author argued that these individuals should not be listed because of the limited nature of their efforts on the manuscript. Our nurse leader colleague suggested writing an acknowledgment for the individuals in question so their contributions would be publicly recognized, but not at the level constituting authorship. This suggestion was met with agreement by the lead authors and the other individuals involved. Our nurse colleague's suggestion provided a practical solution to a sensitive interpersonal situation and was able to bridge the differences of opinion of everyone involved with compassion and respect (see below regarding communication and interpersonal skills).

USE YOUR COMMUNICATION AND INTERPERSONAL SKILLS

Effective leaders apply principles of good communication in their work with individuals and groups. They are clear and direct in their use of language and conveyance of concepts without being brusque or rude. Nurse leader colleagues use language adeptly to convey compassion and concern, yet are firm about a suggestion or direction to be taken. As one nurse leader I work with commented, "I've learned over the years, it is better to be direct with an individual and tell the person 'no' than to dance around the issue."

In providing the "no" (or the "yes"), there is an explanation of the circumstances and logic behind the decision. Nurse leaders are able to discern and acknowledge another individual's perspective through attentive listening and empathic understanding.

FOLLOW THROUGH

As stated earlier in my definition of leadership, leadership involves action. Visionary thinking, strategic planning, and effective communication are critical elements of leadership. When not coupled with action, however, leadership is perceived as ineffective and respect for a leader diminishes. The ability to follow through on tasks, action plans, and even simple communication with others is important when accomplishing a specific project or living the life of a leader. As a nurse leader recently stated to a group of our students, "If others are waiting for you to get something done and you haven't been able to do it, it slows the whole process down." She reflected on a personal experience of a busy time as a student and mother when class work and child demands made it difficult for her to complete a task for a group project quickly. She realized that others in the group were waiting for her before they could move on to their respective responsibilities. As she told the students, this experience provided a valuable lesson in learning the importance of following through on tasks; she shared the lesson with them as a reminder that in group project work, our efforts affect the abilities of others to be able to complete their efforts. Leaders recognize others are waiting for their direction and, at times, completion of a task, for an effort to move forward.

WORK COLLABORATIVELY AND CREATE AN INCLUSIVE ENVIRONMENT

An effective leader draws upon knowledge of group process skills and team work competencies to work collaboratively with others. Creating a working environment, whether in a committee, a department, a unit, or an institutional setting that functions in an open spirit of collaboration, is important for success. A leader who works collaboratively actively seeks, and uses, the input from individuals. There is respect for diversity of perspective and opinion, and a recognition that such diversity frequently comes from having diverse individuals involved, whether such diversity is built upon cultural/ethnic differences, professional backgrounds, skills sets, and so on. While serving on committees chaired by nurses, I observed that there is specific effort on behalf of the nurse leader to address an individual for input in committee discussion if the person has been silent, to summarize the discussion to ensure clarity and/or agreement, and to recognize where differences of opinion exist and to find common ground between them.

Collaboration involves sharing resources, expertise, and seeking to work with others. Our college of nursing has been a leader on our campus with health care simulation. In the plans to build a health care simulation center in the college's building, the college of nursing leadership recognized the value of offering the space to the broader campus and making this valuable instructional environment available to all learners. From this setting, one of our first successful IPE activities was established due to the vision and outstanding collaborative skills of a nurse faculty leader. She worked in partnership with a medical school colleague to design a basic clinical skills (i.e., intubation, venipuncture) teaching workshop to an interprofessional group of medical, nursing, and physician assistant students. The nurse faculty leader applied her knowledge of and passion for health care simulation to include learners from other professions and to team with nonnursing faculty for purposes of developing an outstanding interprofessional learning experience.

A collaborative, inclusive environment arises from multiple elements, such as those stated above, as well as sensitivity to the *subtleties of exclusion*, such as use of language. I observe how my nursing colleagues educate others, including myself, about the use of language and how terms can inadvertently exclude others. My heightened sensitivity to language inclusiveness is due to my nurse leader colleagues. Having worked in a physician-centric environment for most of my professional life, I was unaware of how the term "medical" may be perceived as an exclusive reference to physicians and consequently create a sense of exclusion for other health care professionals. In our planning group for the required interprofessional course, our nursing colleague voiced her concern with the use of "physician" and "nurse" in proposed written vignettes. She suggested we adopt the more inclusive term "health professional," and we all immediately recognized the value of this and agreed to change the term. We appreciated her leadership in fostering a more inclusive and collaborative environment for us and our students through the adoption of inclusive language.

SUMMARY THOUGHTS

Our health care delivery system is demanding increasingly collaborative approaches in the education of future and current professionals, the delivery of patient-centered care, and the engagement of communities to address their health needs. Nurse leaders are intrinsic to the success of these efforts and are changing the future of health in this nation in countless ways. Leadership occurs at multiple levels within any enterprise (and anywhere). It is not merely at the level of the hospital chief executive officer, the college dean, or the nursing unit director, but within committees, patient care teams, and other types of work groups or team efforts. As collaboration becomes more a norm within organizations, leadership should function as a shared capacity among individuals working toward a common goal. Nurse leaders possess valuable professional knowledge and skills, and when coupled with individual talents and strengths, they offer important assets to the success of a collaborative effort. Nurse leaders should recognize how they can best capitalize on their leadership abilities and confidently apply them. We need their voices to improve our collaborative work in transforming health.

4

Leading Change: Perspectives From a University President

Carol A. Cartwright

Commentary
by Joyce J. Fitzpatrick

*C*artwright attributes her own success as a leader
to two major components of her leadership skill
set: communication and collaboration. These are skills
that are important in health care today and serve as a
foundation for excellence in nursing. But even more
basic to effective leadership, in Cartwright's opinion,
is self-knowledge, which comprises understanding
one's own strengths and weaknesses, and building on
one's strengths to identify and achieve realistic goals.
Effective leadership can be taught. Nurse leaders
should be open to new possibilities and value mentorship. Cartwright reflects that leaders surround
themselves with "the best minds." Overall, there is
a lack of confidence among faculty and reluctance
to consider possible benefits of additional leadership
opportunities. Nurse leaders would do well to heed
the advice of Cartwright to build self-knowledge as a
foundation for leadership success.

Another important message of the author is the
need for linking one's own goals with those of the institution in which one works. Thus, leaders must tie their
work to the larger institutional mission and goals, and
effect change in concert with others. This message is

especially important to nurse leaders in health care delivery, as the systems are complexly organized. Although the shared goal of all professionals within health care is to deliver the highest quality care for patients and families, the sheer complexity of the work and the systems challenge health care leaders. Nurse leaders are advised to build on the skills in communication and collaboration that they bring to the table.

Key focus areas: mentor, consensus builder, self-knowledge, collaboration, passionate

I had the privilege of leading two public research universities for nearly two decades (Kent State University from 1991 to 2006 and Bowling Green State University from 2008 to 2011). In these roles, and in the other leadership posts within academe that preceded them, I have witnessed and experienced the inextricable link between personal development and professional progress. In particular, I am convinced of the positive relationship between self-knowledge and the skills needed to embrace, leverage, and lead change. This relationship was not nearly as evident to me as I began navigating a path in higher education. Five decades after beginning that journey, I can affirm that the leadership lessons I have tested and internalized remain applicable to virtually every profession. Because many of the gender stereotypes with which I had to contend have yet to be obliterated, I believe that my experience is of particular relevance to women who hold or aspire to leadership roles.

My selection as Kent State's 10th president gave me the distinction of being that university's first woman president, and the first woman president of a public college or university in Ohio. The path that led me to make history was paved in large measure by the power and empowerment of higher education. Fueled by the can-do attitude instilled in me by my parents, I was the first member of my immediate family to attend college. I earned an undergraduate degree in education (one of the few fields open to women at the time) and took a job teaching first grade. A hunger for further intellectual growth led me to take graduate courses at night. With encouragement from a professor, I applied for and received a federal fellowship for full-time study. Before long, I was immersed in research in the evolving new field of special education. This experience early in my career underscored the importance of being open to new possibilities and the value of mentorship. My leadership path challenges the common perception that successful leaders are born, complete with the requisite temperament and talents. Effective leadership can and should be taught through education and mentorship. In fact, it is via the latter that many of the most critical leadership skills, including listening and relationship building, are transmitted.

Thinking I had found my niche in teaching and research, I accepted a faculty position at The Pennsylvania State University. A colleague who observed me in various meetings noted that I had leadership potential and encouraged an intentional exploration of leadership opportunities. This observation prompted me to consider a different professional path as my faculty career progressed. Having tested the leadership waters in various university committees, when an associate dean position became available, I had the advantages of knowing that I enjoyed the challenges and rewards of leadership, and of being known among my colleagues as a consensus builder. Having reached this first rung of a career ladder in academic administration, I continued to take additional steps as they presented themselves during the succeeding decades, often as the only woman among my immediate circle of colleagues.

In 1990, I agreed to become a candidate for the presidency of Ohio's second-largest public university, knowing that I had the breadth of professional experience and, perhaps most important, the depth of self-knowledge to assume the ultimate leadership post in my field—and to do so at a time of unprecedented challenges in higher education. In the early 1990s, colleges and universities were facing increasing calls for accountability in terms of academic outcomes and fiscal responsibility, pressure to cut costs at a time of growing demand for sophisticated technology tools, the impending retirements of a large cohort of key employees, and a new generation of stakeholders with markedly different needs. These pressures are strikingly similar to those facing today's policy makers, administrators, and other leaders in the health care professions.

Although there was a great deal of interest in me as Ohio's first woman president, the fit between my skills and the institution's needs was sufficiently compelling to soon make gender a nonissue. As I responded to a barrage of requests for media interviews and public appearances during the initial months in office, I did what effective leaders do: directed my energies toward understanding the organization and its culture, and toward finding the optimum balance between leadership and management. As important as it is for leaders to articulate a vibrant vision for their institution or organization, they will not be effective without strong management skills behind the vision. Because effective leadership and effective management are direct correlates, not even the greatest personal charisma can compensate for weak management skills.

Experience also has taught me that effective leaders cannot be effective if they limit communication and collaboration with colleagues in other disciplines or other sectors of the institution. Successful senior administrators function within the organization vertically, as leaders and managers for their portfolio of responsibilities; and horizontally, as experienced critical thinkers and problem solvers, even when issues do not reside in areas for which they are directly responsible. I hold and encourage the view that every leadership role includes opportunities to reach out beyond disciplinary or departmental boundaries for the purpose of finding and cultivating valuable expertise, viable ideas and strategies for improvement, and mutually beneficial partnerships. In complex organizations such as research universities and health care systems, even the most skilled or senior leaders should never convince themselves (or be convinced by others) that they are fully in charge or have all the best answers. Thus, effective leaders surround themselves with the best minds available. I was fortunate that Dr. Greer Glazer, professor and director of parent–child nursing at Kent State, was elected chair of the university's Faculty Senate early in my tenure as president. She served as the point person who worked most closely with me on issues requiring the engagement and support of the faculty.

During Dr. Glazer's 2 years as Faculty Senate chair, we collaborated on a number of fundamental and far-reaching initiatives, including efforts to rethink and redefine faculty scholarship; to build professional-development programs to help faculty incorporate the new wave of teaching and learning tools at their disposal; and to reorganize the university's academic structure, an initiative that affected the future of what was then the School of Nursing. Together, we approached our interactions in a spirit of good faith; with a desire to balance civility with frankness; with the shared goal of moving Kent State considerably farther along the academic–quality continuum; and with a willingness to consider new approaches and paradigms.

As we began our respective leadership roles, campuses nation-wide were beginning to reevaluate the relevance of the "publish or perish" paradigm that was entrenched in American academic cul-ture. This reevaluation was in many ways a result of the publication of *Scholarship Reconsidered: Priorities of the Professoriate* (Boyer, 1990). Ernest Boyer's landmark monograph advocated a broader view of scholarship, one that acknowledged the rich diversity of faculty work at a time when research had eclipsed other forms of scholar-ship (teaching, creative activities, and outreach) in perceived impor-tance. Under this broadened view, all forms of scholarship are held in equal esteem, with *quality* valued over *type* of scholarship. Each category of scholarship was no longer viewed as entailing mutually exclusive intellectual functions. I made it a priority to encourage Kent State's faculty to join the growing national conversation about the definition of scholarship and related issues centered on faculty priorities and productivity. Each of these issues was as politically charged as it was complex.

The plan to spark immediate, widespread discussion of the Boyer model was decidedly risky. At the time, the proposal to dis-card the accepted model had generated serious debate on only a few campuses nationwide. In addition to facing the human ten-dency to resist change, I was asking Kent State's faculty to consider a new mindset as the university was closing in on the long-sought goal of earning Research II status from the Carnegie Foundation for the Advancement of Teaching (the now-revised Carnegie system remains the widely accepted taxonomy of the nation's colleges and universities), a designation that acknowledged faculty strengths in targeted areas of research. Many members of our academic commu-nity already had their eyes fixed on what they deemed to be the even greater prestige of Research I status, which recognized major aca-demic research enterprises. Although I enthusiastically applauded the faculty's significant momentum in basic and applied research, I also observed faculty scholars who were pursuing other types of quality work. I believed that consideration of the Boyer model would be valuable. Further, I knew that Research I status was not a realistic goal for a university at which teaching and undergraduate education played key roles. Even if this had not been my assessment, I was aware that Ohio's legislature was about to mandate that all public universities compile and submit documentation of their efficiency and effectiveness, including detailed accounts of faculty workloads. If we did not proceed with self-assessment, internal planning, and meaningful modifications, externally imposed changes in faculty affairs were inevitable.

It took Dr. Glazer's farsightedness, capacity for thinking out of the box, and, most important, her willingness to take action on behalf of a change in which she saw some merit before significant progress was made in promoting a discussion of a Boyer-based reevaluation of scholarship and related efforts to address legislators' questions about faculty productivity. She made an examination of scholarship a centerpiece of her first term as Faculty Senate chair, supporting a series of open forums based on Boyer's model and creating a Senate Commission on Scholarship. The Commission's thoughtful and sophisticated work in the early 1990s yielded a set of principles for evaluating and rewarding faculty scholarship. These principles became the basis of new tenure and promotion policies that were endorsed by the Faculty Senate and approved by the university's Board of Trustees for implementation in 1997. These defining documents acknowledged the value of all forms of scholarship to the fulfillment of Kent State's multifaceted mission.

Greer Glazer also participated in documenting the broad spectrum of faculty work through personal diaries, a project undertaken in cooperation with the Faculty Senate as part of the aforementioned, state-mandated self-assessment. As a result of that pilot faculty-productivity study, respect for teaching as a full-fledged form of scholarship began to grow across the university, as reflected in the creation of a University Teaching Council to support excellence in college teaching, and the creation of annual awards to recognize the vital contributions of nontenure track and term faculty to the university's teaching mission.

Individually and collectively, these proactive efforts to lead change complemented an institution-wide, strategic-planning initiative, a project that topped my initial list of priorities. Dr. Glazer represented both the Faculty Senate and the School of Nursing as a member of the university's Committee for University Strategic Planning. Her prowess in consensus-building flourished throughout the strategic-planning process, and shined further when university-wide discussions about scholarship and faculty roles expanded to the national stage. Kent State was one of 29 universities invited to participate in the first round of the Pew Higher Education Roundtable project. Supported by the Pew Charitable Trusts, the project enlisted faculty from all disciplines to lead a national dialogue about change in higher education. Greer and I were among the 25 faculty and administrators who formed Kent State's Pew Roundtable. The analysis of change issues provided by the Roundtable remains a model for the kind of thoughtful, inclusive, and respectful dialogue championed by us in our efforts to help our institution and our disciplines navigate into the new millennium.

My work with Professor Glazer was not confined to university-wide issues. Several consequential changes for Kent State's School of Nursing were proposed and debated during the early and middle years of my presidency, leading me to consult with her on a regular basis. The value of working together with equal measures of frankness and respect was reaffirmed as we joined forces to encourage nursing faculty members to envision the transformation of the School of Nursing into a new college. The school's faculty, dean, and other administrators had sought to be designated a College of Nursing for several years. An overwhelming majority contended that standing as a school was tantamount to second-class status, despite the fact that the school was freestanding and had its own dean.

By the mid-1990s, a grassroots, faculty-driven effort to even the organizational playing field had gained sufficient momentum to begin the process of seeking approval from the university's Faculty Senate, Educational Policies Council (EPC), and, ultimately, from the Board of Trustees. With leadership from several senior faculty members, including Drs. Glazer and Karen Budd, and after in-depth discussion at several faculty meetings, the school's Faculty Advisory Council produced a comprehensive memo making the case for the upgrade to college status. Among the most compelling arguments for the change were the facts that the school, which was established in 1970, had evolved into the largest nursing program in Ohio and was in the top 2% in size nationwide; that the name change would be consistent with similar nursing programs statewide and nationwide; that the school was one of only two academic units across the university bearing the name "school"; and that the unit had matured to the point where it made sense to create departments. The document was used by Drs. Glazer and Budd, who had served on the Faculty Senate and EPC, to lobby the Senate's Executive Committee. At the end of the day, they were successful in getting the proposed change on the Senate agenda and in convincing senators and EPC members of the merit of the proposed change.

After working through the required governance and curricular bodies, the Board of Trustees granted college status to the school in 1999. This was a time when the university was endeavoring to create more cohesive academic units. As part of the process toward this goal, I supported the decision to gradually reconfigure a College of Fine and Professional Arts by clustering highly related academic programs and creating smaller and cohesive new colleges or by aligning programs with related programs in existing colleges. As part of this process, we thought that health-related programs (e.g., health education and promotion, and nutrition and dietetics) in the College of Fine and Professional Arts could be assumed by the new College of Nursing.

Having secured recognition as a college and having begun to build a considerable reputation for effective teaching, program development, and innovative research, many within the nursing faculty expressed reluctance to expand the college through the incorporation of additional health care disciplines. They expressed a strong preference for continuing to build on the platform they had created a few years earlier, believing that the proposed expansion might dilute the college's mission, lead to a loss of internal focus, and decrease the college's visibility as the largest nursing program in Ohio. In the end, the proposed reorganization was not enacted and the university opted to align a number of health-related programs within a reconfigured College of Education, Health and Human Services.

Although objections to the proposed reconfiguration were rational, I observed another issue that may have influenced the overall reluctance of the nursing faculty to consider the potential benefits of additional leadership responsibilities: a lack of confidence. In my opinion, this lack of confidence was pervasive enough that it overshadowed the efforts of many among the faculty and administration to advocate the proposed change as an opportunity to create a new, scholarly synergy that could lead to innovative, interdisciplinary research, outreach, and instructional initiatives.

The ensuing years have seen Kent State's College of Nursing build an impressive track record for outstanding scholarship in all its forms. However, this experience points to a leadership lesson that looms large in my experience: At virtually every point in every career, the pursuit of self-knowledge is an endeavor worthy of significant time and effort. The work of achieving self-knowledge comprises several tasks: understanding personal strengths and challenges; articulating personal values and drawing moral "lines in the sand"; and defining personal and professional goals, and charting a realistic course toward their realization. The process of completing these highly personal tasks produces an "internal armor" that creates a capacity to take the calculated risks that almost always precede meaningful change; to accept occasional (and inevitable) miscalculations, to adopt a mindset in which challenges are viewed as potential opportunities, and to proactively and creatively pursue productive partnerships and collaborations. Self-knowledge is a psychological prerequisite for effective leadership in general and for leading change in particular. It is nothing less than essential for current and aspiring nurse leaders who want to help transform health care in ways that benefit society and the nursing profession.

The courage to take well-studied risks was in evidence as the American Association of Colleges of Nursing spearheaded the movement to make the Doctorate in Nursing Practice (DNP) the highest level of preparation for clinical practice. In her capacity as legislative editor for *The Online Journal of Issues in Nursing*, which is based at Kent State, Professor Glazer enlisted me to share thoughts and offer practical advice about the strategic-planning considerations and strong leadership needed for universities to establish the DNP. The resulting article (Cartwright & Reed, 2005) provided an opportunity to work closely with Greer during what would be our last years together at Kent State, and to revisit many of the cultural, political, fiscal, and bureaucratic complexities we had navigated together as part of the process of leading change. Dr. Glazer could have written the article herself. She had been instrumental in developing Kent State's Women's Health Nurse Practitioner program, work that served as a springboard to the many other college- and university-level leadership roles in which she invested so much of herself. Not surprisingly, the article stressed that a highly collaborative approach, one marked by effective communication and a commitment to consensus building, was imperative for enacting a change of this magnitude. Interestingly, writing the article also prompted me to revisit the broadened view of scholarship that Dr. Glazer and I championed more than a decade earlier, as it was apparent that in creating DNP programs, the higher education community would necessarily encourage and accept individuals whose scholarship extends beyond traditional definitions of teaching and research.

The article recounted other basic tenets of leading change, including the imperatives that all leaders and leadership teams act with institutional mission foremost in mind; communicate in word and deed that they support flexible approaches to key issues at hand and on the horizon; and nurture an environment that invites innovation, opting for the possibility of failure rather than clinging to precedents that do not address institutional, community, or societal needs. These beliefs have led me to conceptualize leadership teams as "organizational orchestras" and presidents, chief executive officers (CEOs), and other leaders as their conductors. Each team member is a highly skilled soloist who, at various times in the life of the organization, takes center stage. Although individuals are expected to assume leadership in their areas of expertise, a president, CEO, or other leader has sole responsibility for interpreting a composer's work, orchestrating all parts of a composition into a harmonious whole, and achieving a performance that meets with audience approval. In the public and private sectors alike, the compositions with which we work are mission statements and strategic plans, with audiences ranging from parents to public officials to patients.

Throughout the years, I have also come to view leadership as a responsibility with two, distinct challenges: the "leadership trust" and the "leadership task." The former is to create an environment in which people understand that they have permission, if not an obligation, to participate in the life of their institution or organization; in which they believe that if they get involved, positive change can and will occur. The latter is to ensure that the reality of constant change is understood and that processes for coping with change are in place and being used. Whether the challenge centers on launching new academic programs or changing health care policies, the process of true transformation is a multistep process that must be driven by a clear vision and committed leadership.

I have found a distinction between committed leaders and passionate leaders. I believe that passion for your work, and for the goals toward which you work, is an important part of leadership.

Not only does passion provide personal impetus, it can inspire those around us to pursue their full potential. Having seen Greer Glazer's passion for nursing, commitment to collaboration, and capacity to consider nontraditional views, I was proud to nominate her for a prestigious Robert Wood Johnson Executive Nurse Fellowship. During her term, which spanned 2001 to 2004, I had the additional pleasure of serving as her mentor. The fellowship was an affirmation that Greer had become a consummate leader, possessed of the skills of communication, negotiation, and facilitation that she has continued to employ successfully since becoming dean of the College of Nursing in Health Sciences at the University of Massachusetts Boston in 2004. It is reassuring to know that, nearly 20 years after our leadership paths intersected, she is sharing a wealth of her own leadership lessons with the next generation of nurses and nursing leaders.

REFERENCES

Boyer, E. L. (1990). *Scholarship reconsidered: Priorities of the professoriate.* Princeton, NJ: Carnegie Foundation for the Advancement of Teaching.

Cartwright, C., & Reed, C. (2005, September 30). Policy & planning perspectives for the doctorate in nursing practice: An educational perspective. *Online Journal of Issues in Nursing, 10*(3), Manuscript 6.

A Call to Leadership

Michael F. Collins

Commentary
by Joyce J. Fitzpatrick

*C*ollins begins his remarks on leadership underscoring the importance of higher ideals and a
greater calling among health care professionals. He
cites our privilege to care and our calling and commitment to a life of service as important dimensions of
leadership among health care professionals. As professionals, according to Collins, our primary responsibility is to the ethical nature of our work in the service
of others.

In further delineating the role of professional
nurses as leaders, Collins describes nurses as
(a) patient advocates, underscoring the fact that
each patient needs someone to advocate for them,
particularly in the complexity of today's health care
systems; (b) indispensable team members, participating fully in the team functioning; (c) mentors,
giving and receiving among students of nursing and
with their professional colleagues; and (d) teachers,
of patients and others at all levels. Through these
various roles, all of which are central to nursing,
each nurse has an opportunity to be a leader, for
being a professional nurse is synonymous with being
a leader in Collins's description.

Collins uses a simple story to illustrate this
point: a woman, asking others for help. He expertly
weaves the story of the woman asking for help,

> *"Lady, can you help me?" to illustrate the facets of leadership.* One of the most salient points that Collins makes is that leaders possess an inner peace to respond to the needs of others. This is the expert nurse, whether she or he is providing care and leadership at the local or the global level, whether he or she is a direct care provider, a nurse educator, or a nursing administrator.

Key focus areas: advocacy, privilege to care, code of ethics, collegiality, life of service

"Lady, can you help me?" This was the patient's plaintive cry to the nurses who were hurriedly passing by. "Lady, can you help me?"

The reactions to this simple request were startling. At times, caregivers would stop and hold the patient's hand. Some would simply pass by offering admonitions of: "I'm too busy now"; "I'll be there in a minute, dear"; "You don't need help." Others would say nothing and attribute the patient's request to worsening dementia, senility, or just plain loneliness.

As the patient neared death, all the caregivers stopped to pay their respects. To a person, each reminded the family of a time when the patient stopped them with that familiar line, "Lady, can you help me?" Now, they all expressed their wish that they had stopped to help her once or twice more than they had.

During one such visit, a nurse's aide related how much she loved to care for the patient. When asked what made that experience so special, she stated, "She always said it like it was!" When asked to explain that comment, she elaborated, "I liked her honesty. So many times she would sit in the hall and say, 'Lady, can you help me?' When people told her they were too busy, she would retort, 'You're not too busy! You're lazy!'"

This is a tough but true story. Caregivers who read it will pause to remember when they had a similar experience. It may have been when they walked by a patient in need, observed others do so, or when *they* were a patient, or family member of a patient, in need. No one of us has avoided this situation. Our responses have been varied and, in many cases, underwhelming. However, by exhibiting proper leadership and reaffirming the fundamental covenant between caregiver and patient, we have the ability to improve the patient condition now and into the future.

Such a simple story illustrates such a complex matter. As chancellor of a medical school that benefits from and experiences the unbridled enthusiasm of nursing, medical, and graduate students, there is a constant and consistent imperative to ensure that the education of our students focuses on the human dignity of those for whom it is our privilege to care.

In times past, leadership of schools of medicine and nursing would have directed their efforts to the education of autonomous professionals. Doctors would have memorized *Gray's Anatomy* and biochemical pathways. Nurses would have mastered physiological and pharmacological mechanisms. Educational pursuits were focused on the contents of curricula and the assessment of performance on standardized and licensing examinations.

This is not the case today. Medical and nursing curricula are increasingly competency based, and there is an emphasis on the importance of the practice of our professions within the context of a team of caregivers. Medical and nursing students learn side by side and participate in each other's education and on interprofessional teams. Our educational systems have matured to the point that they focus, in a collaborative professional practice model, on the tenets of our professions and the needs of those we serve. We recognize that it is a privilege for us to care for our patients and not a privilege for our patients to be cared for by us.

Why begin a piece on leadership with a simple story of a woman in need? Clearly, there must be the opportunity to speak of higher ideals or a greater calling. Surely, it would be more pertinent to focus on the leadership abilities needed for successful health care system reform or cost reduction. Definitely, it would be more interesting to cut a path toward the skills essential for increasing access to care or reducing the number of uninsured and under insured in our country. Not so! These are times that call for self-reflection and a recommitment to those for whom we have the privilege to care.

Caregivers in the healing professions are called to a life of service. In the times in which we live, there are less stressful and more lucrative ways to make a living. Yet, we are committed to the values of lifelong learning and the education of those who will succeed us. The hallmark of the health care professions is that our actions are directed by a code of ethics. Different from a vocation, we set aside the realities of the need for gainful employment to a secondary level, as our primary responsibility is to those we serve. When doing so, the leadership skills that are necessary for success in our professions become more clearly elucidated.

There is no higher calling than to accept the responsibility to care for another person. When assuming this obligation, nursing professionals are called to be patient advocates; to acquire a laser-like focus on the patient's needs; to become an indispensable member of a team of professionals who come together to provide care; to educate those professionals who shall join the ranks of the profession; to mentor those in need of example and professional support; to teach patients and colleagues; to adopt a lifestyle with priorities in their proper place; to commit to personal and professional development and quality improvement throughout a career; and to be active participants in the redesign of the health care delivery system. These responsibilities require a myriad of skills and a bundling of resurgent effort. The commitment is as tremendous and important as the benefits of professional practice.

NURSE AS PATIENT ADVOCATE

In the health care setting, be it subacute or acute; inpatient or outpatient; low or high intensity; or community or academic in its orientation, each patient needs advocacy. In the maze that is the American health care system, patients can be lost, both physically and mentally. The patient with a simple request is a perfect example.

"If only as professionals we had the time to care for those in need." This is a call I have heard repeatedly throughout the years. Billions of dollars are spent on alternative medicine options each year, and in many cases patients will explain that they pursued these choices because the practitioner "took the time to sit with me and come to understand my needs." As a result of the frenetic pace of daily practice, health care professionals become immune from the "caring" needs of their patients. Indeed, we have developed "immunity from care" through sheer repetition of our professional practice obligations.

A colleague, for whom I have always held the utmost esteem, was, at all times, present to his patients. Regardless of the time of day or night or the acuity of the situation, this clinician came to the patient when he or she was in need of care. I have observed a similar unyielding commitment to the care of a patient from a number of nursing colleagues that I have had the privilege to work with over the years. No matter what the situation, they had a sense of when a patient needed an extra moment of their caring touch. There was always time to return to administrative responsibilities, but often, there was no second chance to respond to the patient's need of healing. These professionals were present to their patients because they had developed their sense of caring. Patient advocates would not pass by the patient who was calling for their attention.

A FOCUS ON PATIENT NEEDS

A leader possesses the inner peace to respond to the needs of others. Developing the ability to focus intently on the needs of those for whom we care is a learned skill.

It is always affirming to watch a nurse who has developed the ability to assess a clinical situation and to respond in kind. Many times we have heard that a patient's condition improved because a skilled nurse clinician was knowledgeable of the circumstances surrounding the patient's hospital admission or adept at recognizing unexpected turns in that patient's condition. Skilled professionals have that ability to respond when conditions necessitate action.

Many skilled nurses have been accused of being "bossy" or "pushy" because they were insistent that patients receive care when these nurses believed the situation called for it. When focused, such professionals should be viewed as assertive, not as offensively insistent or aggressive. A nurse rapped my knuckles, when, as a student, my hands got a little too close to the surgical field. I still feel the rap and bruise to my ego. But the patient was better for the care and concern this nurse provided. Focused nurse caregivers would respond on the spot to the patient's call for help.

NURSES AS INDISPENSABLE TEAM MEMBERS

The evolution of the caregiving team has been rapid and transformational. Thirty years ago, the attending physician was the all-knowing caregiver whom all others followed. It was their way or the highway; instruments were thrown when they did not get their way; voices were raised when they made their point; and the members of the "team" did what they were told to do.

Today, we see marked change, where the contributions of all team members are welcomed and valued. We recognize that health care is a complex undertaking, and we are confident enough to allow all the members of the care team to fulfill their roles and to practice their profession to the fullest extent of their education, training, and scope. We have come to expect that all caregivers will raise questions when they are concerned that decisions may not be appropriate. In best practice conditions, no longer will there be fear of reprisal for doing so. We are imbued with the belief that all caregivers on the team are conscientious in their commitment to care for the patient and that when there are failures, we look to the system and not to the person to find the root causes.

Like any complex undertaking, the care of a patient is multifaceted and intricate. It is essential that all members of the team participate fully, question always, and commit faithfully. Complete recognition that the care of patients requires interdisciplinary and interprofessional coordination and participation allows patients to be cared for more safely. Autonomous caregivers, in any of the health care professions, have become an outdated modality. The health care team of the present and future would not walk by a patient who called for help.

NURSING EDUCATION

Observing the commitment of nurse educators firsthand is a great benefit of my current leadership responsibilities. There is a serious sense of purpose among committed nurse educators. Their professional standards are fostered in an academic health science center where there is a concentrated focus on students; the education, research, and service missions; and, most important, the patients whose lives will be impacted by their educational experience. Curricular reform efforts are focusing on the competencies needed by skilled nursing professionals at all levels, as well as on the essential underpinnings of a commitment to interprofessional education.

Talented educators become adept at developing their leadership skills. These educators recognize that their students have heightened expectations for the educational expertise and experience they bring to their teaching. Today's nursing students bring varied experiences to their classroom and clinical education sites and are not passive recipients of knowledge. In fact, the active engagement of students and faculty fosters a learning environment that is worthy of those being educated and the profession that they will enter.

At the University of Massachusetts Medical School, there is a principled commitment to interprofessional education. Throughout the nursing curriculum, there are opportunities for students to interact with their graduate and medical student colleagues. Interprofessional clerkships allow nursing students to form teams with their future health care delivery partners, as they pursue learning opportunities in clinical, community, and policy pursuits. Fostering a commitment to interprofessional education establishes the importance of interdisciplinary cooperation and collaboration early in a student's professional life. These skills and values, learned as students enter into practice as collaborators in collegial settings, shall serve them well throughout their professional careers. An interprofessional team learns to respond to patients who call for their help.

NURSES AS MENTORS

Mentoring is an unusual gift: one that is both given and received. Throughout our professional lives, all practitioners benefit from the caring touch of a colleague who extends his or her hand at important moments. Many students look for assistance and advice as they assess whether or not they should embark upon a career as a health care professional and, if so, what direction they should take. During this formative period of a student's life, nurses can play an important role in mentoring students so that they can attain the information necessary for pursuit of their professional dream.

Nursing professionals are held in the highest esteem and revered by their patients. This recognition and the personal satisfaction that comes with the attainment of their professional skills could be better conveyed to those who aspire to careers in nursing. Answering the following questions can help students as they assess the prospects of a career in nursing: Why did you become a nurse? Would you do it again? Are you satisfied as a professional? Can you tell me what you do and how you gain satisfaction from your professional life? Are you able to balance life as a professional with your personal life? Do you think nursing is a good profession? Can you explain your role and responsibilities? Are you an academic? The opportunity to assist those who come behind us as professionals represents an essential responsibility of those who take an oath upon graduation.

The same is true for nurse colleagues. Taking the time to foster colleagues' professional development should be an integral practice of a committed nurse professional. Many in our profession are in need of and benefit from mentoring support and encouragement. Balancing professional responsibilities with life essentials can be demanding. Finding a colleague who will take the time to explore personal and professional hopes and ideals can be a wonderful gift. In order to best care for the patients we serve, we must care for ourselves and those with whom we share professional responsibilities. A good mentor can be a great gift.

Mentoring is fulfilling and requires experience, skill, and commitment in equal measures. Making the time to help a student or colleague can be distracting unless such experiences are viewed as lying at the core of one's professional responsibility. The rewards are satisfying and reflect a generosity of spirit that should be indigenous in the caring professions. A mentor would help a mentee understand the needs of a patient who calls for assistance.

NURSE AS TEACHER

The role of a nurse as teacher is essential to the practice of nursing. Patients who are confronted with an illness, or who wish to maintain their health or improve their healthy behaviors, are in need of education. Patients who receive multiple drugs or varied instructions from a health care provider often find themselves in a quandary when they are alone and must now implement the care plans that they have been provided. Noncompliance is a major factor in patient readmissions and in the failure of treatment regimens. The data are compelling and the response to it underwhelming.

Nurses can play a key role in the education of patients and the improvement of the patient condition. Teaching requires skill. Taking the time to prepare, to clearly explain, and to respond to questions that patients may have requires a commitment to teaching and patience. We must recognize that the complexities of the care setting that we experience as professionals who have become comfortable with the routines of care delivery are often overwhelming to patients. Assessing the needs of each patient as she or he grapples with the care plans she or he has been provided requires a team effort. This may be a responsibility for which the nurse becomes the captain of the team. Teachers would recognize the needs of patients who call for their assistance.

COMMITMENT TO PROFESSIONAL DEVELOPMENT

Membership in the health care professions requires a commitment to lifelong learning. On the day I graduated from medical school, there was only one paper published on the yet unexplained pneumonias in immunocompromised men in San Francisco. It hardly seems that long ago, and yet, had my education stopped then, I would not have been able to care for patients with HIV.

All health care professionals must commit to furthering their knowledge and to keeping current with their educational pursuits. The responsibility to care for others requires nothing less.

In the health education fields we commit to providing education for a lifetime. As educators and professionals, we must redouble our efforts to fulfill that commitment. The complexity of the health care professions necessitates that imperative. With the development of experiential learning through simulation and standardized patient experiences, lifelong learning can be creative and challenging. The skill to commit to this endeavor must permeate our professions.

Lifelong learners would know to respond to a patient's call for assistance. Outstanding nurse leaders respond to these principles. They exude confidence and competence, which are balanced by humility and commitment. In the interactions with their colleagues and with other professionals on the health care team, they guide the actions of the team toward quality and an unwavering commitment to the patient. There is no compromise when it comes to best practice patterns, the evaluation of data, and the implementation of care plans. Respect is given and expected and deserved in turn. Collegiality is a hallmark of professional relationships.

There is no question that the complexity of health care delivery into the future will call on these leadership skills and necessitate heightened attention to their development. On the most successful teams, there is full appreciation of the skills of each participant and a respect for the suppression of egos that foster the success of the team as an enterprise. Nurse leaders have a unique opportunity to leverage their professional knowledge and expertise to bring health care team performance to greater levels. The focus on the patient and the advocacy that the patient feels from the nurse uniquely position nurse leaders for this opportunity.

Over the past 2 years, the Institute of Medicine and others have identified opportunities for nurses to expand their advocacy efforts, including the call for active participation in the redesign of the health care delivery system. Nurse leaders, as integral members of the patient care team, need to work in partnership with other health care professionals to design the health care delivery system of the future. Such a partnership requires that nurse leaders be integral to efforts in which strategy and policy related to heath care are discussed, debated, and determined.

Nurse leaders should be duly represented at the highest management and board levels to appropriately reflect the critical importance of nursing to the health care delivery system of the future. Let us return to the patient whose story began this journey into leadership skills and expectations.

There is greater awareness in today's health care milieu that patients often become forgotten in the health care system. There is a drive toward technological innovation and best practice development. The focus on quality is receiving increased attention by leaders of all professional disciplines. Payers are losing patience with the inability to reduce costs and the needs of the uninsured are the fodder for intense political debate.

But the patient still needs our care and attention. The best leaders in our professions are able to overcome the tendency to become lulled into complacency as we see a large volume of patients. Our personal defense mechanisms afford us the ability to become detached, even if ever so slightly, from the constant and consistent needs of our patients. Entry into, care within, and discharge from health care offices and facilities can be disorienting and disabling for patients and their families. Our ability to recognize this reality is a skill that all professionals must continue to hone.

Frequently, patients ask for a moment of our time. They want to feel and know that they have our undivided and unhurried attention. This does not seem too much to ask, but it is most difficult to accomplish and fulfill.

I chose a simple story to make a complex point. I could have placed the patient in a more acute setting, but the situation might have become the excuse for the behavior. In each instance in which we care for a patient, we should assure that our actions are oriented to a promotion of human dignity for our patients. This is a high calling and most suitable to the professions that we have chosen.

Time and again, leaders are confronted with the complaint that "you would never have allowed your mother to be treated this way." In responding to these situations, we choose to remove the personal reference and to focus on the details of the encounter. We strive to advocate, focus, educate, teach, mentor, collaborate, and continue our professional development. In doing so, we lead and improve the care of those entrusted into our hands.

In this instance, the patient who asked, "Lady, can you help me?" was my mother. How would you respond?

Lessons Learned From the Nurse in Charge

Arthur G. Cosby

Commentary
by Joyce J. Fitzpatrick

In sharing his perspective on nursing leadership, Cosby writes about an invisible star in the profession, one whose views of nursing and humanity had a profound effect not just on the author but on others whose lives she touched. Cosby's mother, the nurse leader he writes about, taught lessons of leadership and responsibility and believed that there was greatness in teaching others and in improving their lives through health care.

Cosby believes leaders must be ethical, understanding the far-reaching consequences of their actions. He also shares the importance of symbolism as an important characteristic of leaders. This is a timely and noteworthy statement as nurse leaders and nurses everywhere often struggle with the image they want to project. Leaders must inspire confidence in the manner in which they present themselves. They must clearly communicate that they are in charge. This requires discipline in presentation at all levels. The leader is not the confidant of the followers, but is in a different collegial relationship. The leader must stand out, and it must be clear that she or he is disciplined in thought and deed. As Cosby describes, leadership discipline is an essential component. In his summary Cosby identifies the importance

*of integrity, compassion, responsibility to others,
discipline, and a sense of humanity as the essential
characteristics of leaders.*

Key focus areas: discipline, consequences of action, influence,
risk taking, self-knowledge

In our universe there are many different kinds of stars. Some, such
as the supernova, emit a great deal of light, are easy to see, and
clearly display their prominence to all. By definition, supernovas
are "extremely luminous" and can briefly outshine the entire gal-
axy. At the same time, there are invisible stars that are more difficult
for us to see. They are sometimes embedded within a large group
of stars, their light obstructed from view by others. Some invisible
stars are so incredibly powerful that their gravity does not allow
light to escape. In the cosmos of American medicine, we have many
stars, and more often than not, we find constellations of supernova
physicians surrounded by less visible nursing stars.

Astronomers tell us that invisible stars are not really invisible,
but rather, they are only invisible if we do not know how to look
for them. I believe the same is true for many stars of the nursing
profession. Sometimes the most influential, effective, and impactful
are not recognized for their true greatness. In this chapter, I want to
write about one nurse who was a star in her profession, sometimes
an invisible star, but always a supernova to me.

You see, my mother was a *nurse* in every way, and she made
sure that the significance of nursing was not lost on me. Her perspective on nursing, the practice of her profession, and her view
of humanity shone brightly and truly had a profound effect on my
life. My mother, the nurse, led me to understand what constitutes
leadership, my responsibilities to others, and very significantly, the
role of women in the modern world.

Lillie Mae McIntire Cosby, some called her Mac, was born
100 years ago in a much different place and time. The hills of
Kentucky were a hard life for many. Small farms, subsistence agri-
culture, large families, physical isolation, and poverty were widespread. She was 1 of 11 children and was hardly a child of privilege;

her parents were tenant farmers of modest means. In spite of numerous obstacles, Mac and her older brother finished high school. He went off to college, and she went to nursing school at Nashville General Hospital. They were to become part of "the greatest generation," the generation who endured the Depression, won World War II, and helped create prosperity for the nation at large.

Mac graduated from nursing school during the Depression. Her first job was working as a public health nurse in the very rural and isolated region around Oakridge, Tennessee. From the stories she told, this was truly difficult work. Her home visits were sometimes by horseback, sometimes by buggy, and sometimes by automobile. Health literacy was low, and health care was, at best, limited. But there was an upside. The chance to make a difference and to contribute was ever present. She always communicated that, in spite of these hardships, there was also great personal satisfaction in improving the lives of others and the sense of accomplishment that brought. When I recall the stories my mother told, there was more often than not a lesson for me, and usually it was an important lesson that I needed to learn. I loved her stories and always listened carefully.

After a year or so, Mac moved back to Kentucky and was, for over a decade, the only registered nurse practicing in her county. Interestingly, there were usually more doctors than registered nurses in the Depression-era hill country. Sometime after returning, she married my father, who was a much older country doctor, and theirs was a "May–December" marriage—her first and his second. The marriage produced two children, my brother and me.

My father had a well-established practice, and with the marriage, Mac effectively became part of it. She took on the major task of getting his books in order, his patient accounts up to date, and, I suppose, imposing a rational accounting system on a Depression-era medical practice. This was no small effort because a great deal of my father's practice was based on the barter system: farm commodities for medical services. He was paid in chickens, vegetables, labor, and even moonshine whiskey. To prove her worth, my mother began contacting patients to bring delinquent accounts current. One of Dad's long-time patients was over a year behind in payments. When contacted by Mac, he asked her if she was willing to take a milk cow to settle the account. Mac thought that a milk cow was better than a delinquent account and that the patient had offered a good deal. She accepted Betsy as an account paid-in-full.

That same day, the cow was delivered, and Mom had the farmer put Betsy in the field behind the family home.

When Dad returned from a home visit, he immediately wanted to know whose cow was in his pasture and why it was there. Mac proudly told him of her success in settling an account that would not have been paid otherwise and fully expected a compliment for her good work. To her surprise, Dad's immediate response was, "Mac, do you know what you have done? You have taken their only milk cow. The children will have no milk and will be hungry and probably sick! Make sure that cow gets back to them immediately." The cow was returned that very afternoon.

My mother loved to tell this story. It was clearly self-deprecating humor, and it also conveyed a powerful moral message. This story, to me, appropriately extended the ethical principle of "first do no harm," beyond the immediate medical procedure, to more global consequences for the overall well-being of individuals, their families, and by extension, the community. I believe effective leaders must have the same generalized ethical concerns that extend beyond the immediate settings of their actions. Leaders need to know the far-reaching consequences of their actions and care about those who are affected.

By their very nature, the rural settings in which Mac and my father practiced medicine created challenges for all those in the health care field. Isolation and limited transportation required much of their work to be carried out through home visits. The small population base in rural Kentucky simply could not support a high degree of medical specialization, and the few existing health care providers had to become generalists. As they practiced in rural counties with no hospitals, infant deliveries were most often performed at home.

Mac was especially proud of the large numbers of babies she delivered, and I was always fascinated by her accounts of home deliveries. The standard protocol was for Mac and my father to go to the home when the mother went into labor and stay with the family until the child was born. This of course resulted in many lengthy home visits. It also resulted in doctors and nurses knowing a great deal more about the everyday lives of their patients.

In keeping with household gender roles at the time, Mac would typically stay with the expectant mother and carry out the delivery, while my dad and the expectant father would talk in the front room and often share whiskey, usually moonshine. There was clearly a different legal climate for malpractice. My father would typically not get involved with the delivery unless a serious complication arose. This was actually fortunate training for my mother because later she would perform a similar role when the rural counties built their first hospitals, and she worked for them. The small, rural hospitals normally had few doctors, and usually they were only on call. As the head nurse, she routinely delivered babies when the doctors were not able to get there on time. She used to estimate that she had delivered over 500 babies by herself during home visits and at the small hospitals.

To me, this was in many ways pioneering work that helped define the range of roles that nurses now occupy. The necessity of her, and nurses like her, delivering medical services with such a great deal of autonomy helped set the stage for a high level of specialization and focused expertise. Her stories about delivering babies really brought home to me the great significance of her work and the responsibility and risk taking that was involved in providing health care in extremely difficult conditions. To me, leadership that makes a difference more often than not involves these very important features. The type of risks that I have encountered in my own work pales in comparison with the risks associated with home deliveries and other types of health care that she provided on a daily basis. Still, her experiences helped shape my approach to risk taking and decision making.

A year after the end of World War II, things changed abruptly for our family. As you may recall, my father was much older than my mother and quite senior to be starting a second family. One morning while he and Mac were getting ready for the day, he suffered a massive and fatal heart attack, leaving my mother with two preschool boys to raise.

His death marked the end of the medical practice they had enjoyed. The family estate was divided between the children of both marriages and Mac. In the end, there was relatively little wealth to share. Mac was on her own with two young children, and it would be the nursing profession that provided for the family.

At about the same time of my father's death, the county opened its first hospital, and Mac was recruited to be both the hospital administrator and the head nurse. Today it is difficult to imagine that anyone would hold both of these positions, even in a small rural hospital. These were clearly positions of great responsibility and of great significance to the people of the county. At the time, I was too young to fully appreciate how unusual this was and how much respect they had for Mac to entrust her with such responsibility.

The memory of her in this role is vivid in so many ways. My recollections of my mother, head nurse, are rooted not only in the visual image but also in her speech and even the sound she made travelling the hospital halls. There was a distinctive whoosh made with every step of her brisk walk and heavily starched uniform. You could not only see her coming, you could hear her coming. My mother had a very clear image of how a nurse should look, and there was no doubt to anyone who met her that Mac was a nurse, and indeed, a serious nurse. The uniform was starched, the shoes were shined, and the back was straight. She clearly understood there was symbolism associated with leadership, and she knew exactly how to convey to others that she was not only a nurse, but the nurse in charge.

In my mother's mind, discipline was a critical aspect of good health care. As head nurse, she supervised a large number of junior nurses, aids and orderlies, many of whom had limited formal health care training. At the start of each shift, my mother would line up the nurses and aids for inspection. Her inspections were every bit as tough as those I later experienced in the military. You simply would not work in her hospital unless your uniform was cleaned and starched, your shoes shined, your hair properly groomed, and most important, your hands and fingernails clean. She was very serious about the spread of germs in hospitals and saw discipline and cleanliness as a fundamental aspect of health care. She would tell me that no one would want to be touched by someone with dirty hands and fingernails, and that touching patients was an important part of health care. To her, discipline was an absolutely essential part of leadership. It was not only that the leader herself needed self-discipline but that, through her leadership, she encouraged and instilled discipline in those whom she led.

Frankly, discipline is not my strong suit, but I have little doubt that the lessons conveyed through my mother's practice of nursing moved me substantially toward a more disciplined life than I would have achieved without her influence. Few worthy things can be accomplished without the exercise of discipline, and the lack of discipline can lead to very unfortunate results.

About the time I was completing elementary school, things changed once again for our family. Mac accepted an offer to become the school nurse at Columbia Military Academy in Tennessee. She moved from her home in Kentucky to the military school, sacrificing her family and friends, so that my brother and I would have the experiences, opportunities, and advantages afforded by an academy that we would never have had in the rural public schools.

Columbia was a boys' boarding school with a strong academic and military tradition. It could not have been more different from the public schools in rural Kentucky. The school was very expensive, and the students were from mostly affluent backgrounds. The cadets came from various regions of the United States and from a number of foreign countries. The school hospital was located in the center of the campus and became our family home. The boarding school also had a much different environment in that it provided total immersion in an educational institution. My life was highly structured; everything was scheduled and announced by bugle call.

I believe that the school nurse job was the easiest position that my mother ever held. The cadets were generally healthy, and rarely would she have to be involved with severe medical issues. Colds, cuts, and bruises were the big issues at morning sick call. School athletics occasionally produced a few broken bones. The hospital had a ward and a couple of private rooms, but rarely were there any cadets in the hospital.

For the years we were at Columbia, my mother's responsibilities were more relaxed, and she adapted well to the pace of a boys' boarding school. This gave me time to learn more things from my mother. She was an avid reader of almost everything: newspapers, magazines, and books were everywhere in our home. Fortunately, some of this rubbed off on me, especially an interest in current affairs and politics. Also, she put me in an environment in which there were many male role models. Most of my teachers were men; my coaches were men; and of course, the boarding cadets were all male. There is little doubt that my mother's sacrifices produced a life-changing event that would have profound consequences on my worldview, my ambitions, and ultimately, the modest successes I have enjoyed. Mac moved us to the military school primarily as my mother, but she could not have done it had she not been a nurse.

It was very important to me that I had a mother who could do so many things and do them well. Not only was she a mother and nurturer, she was also a woman who was the breadwinner, who could successfully carry out most any job—even the most difficult. Over the course of her career, she actively carried out the health care responsibilities of head nurse, hospital administrator, emergency room nurse, physician's assistant, obstetrics nurse, public health nurse, school nurse, nurse practitioner, and probably a number of other roles of which I am unaware. My concept of women's roles must have been shaped at a very early age in ways unconventional for the times. I do not believe that I ever wondered about the ability of women to lead and accept the most demanding and responsible positions. Interestingly, this was so ingrained in my worldview that I did not understand she had given me this special gift until the conversations of the women's movement had gained momentum years later. It was a gift that would later give me a tremendous advantage as a leader.

After my brother and I left the military school for college, Mac returned to her hometown in Kentucky to take care of her aging mother. She once again worked as a head nurse until her retirement. I became a university professor and administrator and worked throughout the South—in Mississippi, Louisiana, and Texas.

In my university work, there have often been biases about the role of women in academia, and early in my career, there were many university women who were institutionally limited in their ability to achieve. It was not simply that institutions were not recruiting women. When women were hired, they were not given the same opportunity and expectations for achievement that was afforded their male colleagues. Looking for talent early on as a department head, and more recently as a research center director, it quickly occurred to me that there was a substantial group of talented professors who were being underutilized. I knew that if I could recruit them and give them an environment that did not limit their abilities, wonderful things would happen.

My research center has, for over 25 years, grown and flourished at a rate that exceeds most similar organizations on campus, and it compares quite favorably nationally. It is a place where women and men can excel, and our growth, compared with other organizations, can directly be tied to the success of women. My mother gave me a competitive advantage as a university administrator because I was so accustomed to her success and achievements that I was better equipped to recognize the talent of women and include their recruitment as a critical aspect of developing a research organization.

Although my mother and I were physically separated because of my university appointments, we remained close and shared our experiences and interests through the years. A few years after her retirement, both Mac and my grandmother died within 2 weeks of each other. Of course I always loved my mother, and because of her success and accomplishments as a nurse, I also respected and admired her as a professional woman who could do miraculous things. The opportunity to write this chapter on nursing and leadership has allowed me to organize my thoughts and more fully appreciate how incredible she really was. As you can tell from my earlier comments, Mac had a great influence on me, personally and professionally. She gave me a sense of integrity, compassion, responsibility to others, discipline, and a general view of humanity that has served me well in leadership positions. I had the good fortune of learning by example from a true supernova.

7

An Economist's Perspective on Nurse Research Leadership

Jerry Cromwell

Commentary
by Joyce J. Fitzpatrick

*C*romwell has a rich history of both preparing nurse leaders in research and collaborating with nurse researchers. On the basis of his extensive experience, he offers cogent advice on leadership roles that nurses can fill in research on health care policy formulation and implementation that will change the course of health care payment, delivery, and quality throughout the United States. Importantly, his exploration into potential leadership roles for nurses begins with a wide view on the vast array of opportunities for nurse researchers not merely to sit at the policy table, but to shape the discussions and the solutions to vexing health care problems. Cromwell believes that nurse researchers can provide leadership through the development of skills in management, program development, research, and teaching. He asserts that leadership qualities can be developed over time, and that as one develops these skills, it is important to "pass on the torch" to the next generation of students and potential leaders. Thus, the role of the leader as teacher is critical.

To illustrate the characteristics of nurse research leaders, Cromwell describes one such leader with whom he has worked for more than two decades.

He details her skills in project leadership, her technical research skills, and her management skills. In addition, he describes her leadership style as that of a "doer," focused on getting things done, with extraordinary intensity, and leading by example. From this nurse leader, he describes many lessons learned, including the need for a strong work ethic, the ability to see the "big picture," the need for attention to detail, and strong communication skills. Cromwell also identifies other nurse researchers who are leading policy development at the government levels, including those at some of the top federal agencies. Cromwell's two most important messages for aspiring nurse leaders are knowledge is power and there is room at the table for those who possess the knowledge.

Key focus areas: technical skills, teacher, public policy skills, problem solver

The asymmetric physician–nurse relationship in direct patient care, traditionally, has been one of leader (physician) and subordinate (nurse). As captain of the ship, the physician has exercised the broadest scope of practice in practicing *medicine* and is responsible for admitting and discharging patients, performing operations, writing prescriptions, diagnosing and recommending treatment, and managing almost all of the hospital's clinical services. By contrast, only advanced practice nurses have performed these activities and, in most states in collaboration with physicians. *Nursing* has most often been relegated to carrying out the physician's orders. Taking on "life-or-death" responsibilities naturally prepares medical students to be leaders. Nurses are not asked to make independent decisions with major health implications, and to this day the Medicare program requires that all nurses, in their daily activities, be under a physician's supervision. This arrangement is highly efficient. Tasks are performed depending upon breadth and depth of training with corresponding higher and lower incomes for physicians and nurses, respectively. An unfortunate byproduct of this arrangement, however, is the stunted growth in nurses' critical thinking. Left with the execution of physicians' orders, nurses deliver medications with predetermined and prepackaged doses, follow protocols, take notes on patients' progress for physicians' review, and attend to patients' bodily needs. Although many nurses make their own "diagnoses" of patients' problems—it is only human nature given their didactic training, they also know better not to share them with their patients.

When I began teaching health economics to nurses in the PhD program at the University of Massachusetts Boston 4 years ago, I was struck with their general lack of self-confidence. When, in course discussion, I learned that many students filled senior management roles at major teaching institutions (more later) or public policy agencies, I was even more baffled by their reticence and difficulty in learning what I thought were fairly simple economic principles. Often, I heard students moan, "I'm no good at math. I can't draw and explain graphs very well." I knew my students were inherently intelligent. How else could they complete rigorous nurse training courses, complete master's degrees, and manage nursing floors or entire hospital nurse staffs? Most frustrating of all was their hesitancy to strike out on their own intellectually, to criticize a body of literature, a psychometric scale, or an "accepted way" of thinking of a social process. "I can't do that," they said. "There is no literature using this approach," or "that is not the way it is usually done in the literature." Yet, in our program, they are not being prepared as nurse practitioners, but rather as health service researchers. A good researcher must exercise a critical mind, accept nothing at face value, and question received wisdom. Doctoral students must be willing to learn at least two new, nonclinical languages, the language of math and statistics, and how to "talk" to the computer. They must be able to succinctly capture social processes in a few well-chosen words, often best explicated using mathematical symbols. Even more challenging, nurse researchers must step off their nursing floors, away from individual patients, and learn to describe how whole systems work. How might the hospital industry respond to financial penalties for complications? How might a low-income community respond to an innovative cardiovascular educational program? How many nurse practitioners will be needed in 10 years as medical students continue to opt out of primary care? Trained to follow routinized protocols and clinical pathways, many nurses I have encountered in the classroom struggle to remember their ninth-grade algebra, Cartesian graphing, and thinking about how x affects y, when x is a new drug rehabilitation program and not an antibiotic, and y is life years saved and not simply redness from infection.

It does not take a PhD economist, however, to see that a new order is coming. Health care costs have escalated to the point that not only most citizens but whole governments cannot afford to pay for proper health care. Among physicians, a slow migration over 30 years has taken place away from poorer paying primary care to technical and invasive specialties. Yet, more recently, payers, clinicians, researchers, and even politicians, despite refusing to enact serious workforce planning, have lamented the lack of primary care physicians in America to coordinate fractionated care for the chronically ill. Not nearly enough is being done one-on-one to change patients' unhealthy lifestyles and avoid expensive interventions after it is too late. Nurses are best suited to fit the growing gap. They have most of the necessary training. They are much less costly to train than specialized physicians. Nevertheless, some nurses still need to lead outside the office, to plan and mobilize resources at the state and national levels.

As a teacher, this is where I come in. I have three broad goals for this chapter. First, I intend to review the range of roles that nurses can fill with special emphasis on research leadership in policy formulation and implementation. Second, I will provide two examples of research leadership, one based on a single nurse doing technical health research at the highest level, and another characterizing the activities and skills required of PhD nurses working in the Centers for Medicare & Medicaid Services (CMS) in Washington, DC. These nurse leaders do not teach new nurses. They do not replace primary care physicians. Rather, they change the course of health care payment, delivery, and quality throughout America. I conclude with a few heartening examples of fledgling researchers in our own program.

NURSING CAREERS

Figure 7.1 shows the range of employment and leadership opportunities open to nurses in either the private sector or government. The vast majority of nurses provide patient care in hospitals,

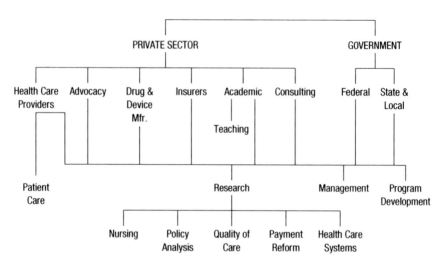

FIGURE 7.1
Range of employment and leadership opportunities for nurses.

clinics, nursing homes, and so on. In the private sector, others work in their own associations (e.g., American Nursing Association [ANA], American Association of Nurse Anesthetists [AANA]) or advocacy groups (e.g., American Association of Retired Persons [AARP], American Cancer Society [ACS]). Others work for drug and device manufacturers, the Pharmaceutical Research and Manufacturers of America (PhRMA), or insurers (e.g., Blue Cross/Blue Shield, Kaiser). Many work in academic institutions teaching and doing research. Finally, a substantial number work for consulting organizations such as Rand, Mathematica Policy Research (MPR), the Urban Institute, as well as where I do my health economics research, the Research Triangle Institute (RTI). Many nurses also work for federal, state, and local governments, including the Agency for Healthcare Research and Quality (AHRQ), the Centers for Disease Control (CDC), the CMS, and the National Institutes of Health (NIH), along with state health departments.

Besides their traditional role of caring for patients, nurses teach other nurses in colleges of nursing, and in their government capacity, they develop new programs in public health and service payment and delivery. Nurses in all settings also fill management or research roles. Administrative roles range from managing a cardiovascular unit of a hospital or neighborhood health clinic to directing a federal research division of the CDC or a college of nursing. As for research, I have categorized their activities into five broad areas:

1. Nursing
2. Policy analysis
3. Quality of care
4. Payment reform
5. Health care systems

The majority of research nurses focus on developing evidence-based methods for improving nursing care, mostly in academic settings. Nurses working in government, advocacy groups, and in consulting usually conduct policy analyses of changes in health care payments and regulations. Policy analysis is the science of reviewing and summarizing extant research in order to formulate and evaluate policy options. The remaining three research areas I call "basic health services research." Master's and PhD nurses work in government agencies developing and testing measures of quality, conducting comparative effectiveness analyses, and in developing complex surveys on patient satisfaction. Nurses in drug and device companies are involved in clinical trials evaluating health outcomes from new interventions. Highly trained nurses also work in multidisciplinary teams designing and evaluating payment reforms and in understanding how health care systems respond to various incentives and environmental changes.

What does it take to be a leader? Hundreds of books have been written on the subject and many fortunes made on the lecture circuit. Leadership qualities are no different in the many nursing roles versus other professions; only the degree of emphasis varies. Let me begin with management.

Management

Consider the qualities of a good nurse manager—a leader of people. This is a leader with strong interpersonal skills, a person who is sensitive to how new ideas and rules are presented and to how individuals accept direction and respond to criticism. They are excellent at motivating others and adept at when to delegate and to whom. A management leader is remarkably tolerant of bureaucratic rules and regulations, a person who thrives under time pressure and takes pleasure in sharing in team accomplishments. A good manager is highly organized, sets clear priorities, and is flexible in responding to changes in the external environment. Although never comfortable in chaotic situations, a management leader—through straight thinking and the "force of personality"—takes responsibility and leads his or her staff with assurance to calmer waters. This manager can also cope with leading staff one minute and reporting to superiors the next. A team-building leader is both a team leader and an integral part of a larger organizational "team."

Program Development

A nurse leader in the public (and occasionally the private) sector is sometimes responsible for developing and implementing a new program. It might be a rapid response initiative to a flu outbreak, a cardiovascular education program, or a new way of paying for higher quality care. Most of the necessary management skills are necessary here, but often under less chaotic, time-sensitive conditions. This leader derives more pleasure than other managers from understanding and making systems work better. Groups, not particular individuals, are mostly the focus. An effective program leader is one who relishes synthesizing research and substantive knowledge to form a new policy. Ultimate success, though, requires perseverance and an unusually high tolerance level for bureaucratic and political in-fighting. Primary gratification comes from helping individuals "from afar" and over time without the immediate feedback enjoyed by managers of clinical staffs.

Research

A leader of research may have management and program development skills, but these traits are generally not essential to a successful research career. Absolutely essential in leading successful research is critical thinking and technical superiority. A productive researcher must have a skeptical mind and a love of solving puzzles. Above all, a research leader, first, is a good scientist who takes little on faith, is curious, and, like many youngsters, loves to "take things apart" to see what makes them work. The researcher is skeptical of the conventional wisdom and is not afraid to criticize established theories and authorities, including physicians and highly published authors. The best leaders are intellectual risk takers.

They see new ways of looking at old problems and make substantial investments of their time and reputation to correct flaws in our understanding of underlying causal forces.[1] In these endeavors, they are extraordinarily persistent.

Equally important are their technical skills. Researchers, to be leaders, must command high respect for their breadth and depth of knowledge regarding research methods, theory, and statistics. Theories will differ depending upon subject area, but nurse leaders, at a minimum, must be well grounded in clinical knowledge (e.g., physiopathology, diagnostic assessment, medications). No nursing leader can work with physicians, which they inevitably must, without speaking and thinking the same language. Still, they should bring more to their work. They must be conversant with one or more interdisciplinary fields such as sociology, psychology, political science, or economics. Their research usually addresses the human condition beyond the human body. Leading research on health policy, quality, and payment reforms requires familiarity with organizational theory, psychometrics, epidemiology, cost-effectiveness, and theoretical constructs based on provider supply and patient demand. Leaders also evince a working knowledge of statistical methods, including sample design, hypothesis testing, and power and regression analysis. Although nurse leaders may not know complex statistical sampling and analytic methods such as maximum likelihood estimation, they must be able to direct statisticians and interpret complex quantitative results. They must be able to design qualitative studies, conduct interviews, and quickly recognize threats to internal and external validity in study designs, legislated coverage, and payment mandates. True research leaders put it all together, taking classroom concepts and applying them successfully to practical questions.

Effective researchers need not have the interpersonal skills of managers nor their desire to work in large teams. Some may be good mentors and show less experienced researchers "how to do it." Others simply take a "learning by doing" approach: "Watch me, do like me, keep up with me." They may not "suffer fools gladly" like managers and team players and tend to be impatient with

---

[1] The ultimate risk taker brings to mind Albert Einstein, who spent a decade of his most productive research career trying to prove that heavenly bodies did not attract each other, as Newton thought; instead, they simply "curved" space in around them and caused massless light to bend and time itself, to slow down.

unfocused, naive, thinking. They still may be effective research leaders, nonetheless, through their written publications and oral presentations. They can be the "rainmakers" who provide younger researchers with the financial support to gain research experience. Great researchers do not have to be loved.

Teaching

Good teachers naturally have the mind of a researcher. Like researchers, teachers must be curious problem solvers. Critical thinking is also required. A good teacher must truly understand the logic, the mathematics, and the statistics of the subject matter to present it in the most succinct, intuitive way. Ideally, they are active researchers themselves. By doing research, teachers are more sensitive to the assumptions, challenges, and limitations of the theories and methods they impart to students. Using their own research as examples also reinforces their authority on, and commitment to, a topic.

Unlike many researchers, however, leading teachers must be mentors at heart. They must derive pleasure from sharing theories and methods with others—especially those who are eager to learn but lack the necessary skills in research design, clinical or program operations, and mathematics. To do this well requires a combination of strong technical skills and an extroverted personality. Humor always helps. Nobody likes to learn from a robot. The material can be dry enough. Researchers need to be available to students, must be patient, and never abandon students as long as they are trying. Leaders push students, expecting a bit more than the students think they are capable of doing. Learning half of a lot is better than learning most of a little. Complete command of each topic is unreasonable to expect, but once exposed, students can at least more critically evaluate what they read and what comprehensive research is all about. Exposing willing minds to new ideas and methods is a noble, often selfless, act.

Summary

No one becomes a great leader (or athlete) overnight. No one is born a great leader. Yes, genetic material and early childhood experiences shape people's personalities and make them more inclined to be good team-building managers, good teachers, or "ivy-tower" researchers. Leadership qualities, though, come through accumulated experience with a dose of natural selection. Good researchers can become great managers by marrying previously developed technical skills with a collaborative temperament. Some researchers can embrace program development if they are willing to deal with the social and political obstacles facing enactment and implementation.

Let me now provide an example of a nurse who abandoned a successful clinical nursing career in a major Boston teaching hospital to become a true research leader.

NANCY McCALL, RN, SCD

Roughly 20 years ago, I hired Nancy as a senior researcher in our company, Health Economics Research (HER). She had a master's degree in nursing from Purdue's College of Nursing and was working in Washington at the Health Care Financing Administration (HCFA) while finishing her PhD thesis at the Harvard School of Public Health. Before returning to graduate school, Nancy had worked for several years as a cardiac critical care nurse at Brigham & Women's Hospital in Boston. Her Harvard curriculum was novel, especially for a nurse. It required her to take courses in graduate microeconomics in the economics department where she applied calculus, statistics, and regression methods to theories explaining consumer and corporate behavior. Eventually, she completed her thesis with Joe Newhouse, the program director and former chair of the Medicare Prospective Payment Assessment Commission (MedPAC). Her research tested theoretical predictions of physician responses to fee freezes on costly procedures in the late 1980s. During her 2 years at HCFA, she was one of many government project officers (POs) overseeing HER projects and writing federal Medicare rules and regulations. After HER was sold to nonprofit RTI in 2002, Nancy has continued to manage projects and contribute to institute management. She is a truly extraordinary leader of fellow researchers.

Project Leadership

Over Nancy's career, she has led 15 to 20 multidisciplinary, multimillion dollar federal projects and been a coinvestigator on many others. She is currently Project Director (identical to Principal

Investigator on government grants) on six projects simultaneously, including the following:

- Medicare's High Cost Chronic Care Demonstration
- Evaluation of Hospital Responses to Congress' Hospital Acquired Condition (HAC) Legislation
- Tricare's Disease Management (DM) Evaluation
- Evaluation of Medicare's Medical Home Evaluation
- Medicare's Acute Care (Hospital) Episode Demonstration
- MedPAC's Assessment of Data to Correct Flaws in Medicare's Physician Fee Schedule (PFS)

Together, these projects involve more than ten PhD researchers and $15 million. Her project team also recently completed a 5-year congressionally mandated evaluation of the Medicare Health Support Pilot Program that determined the cost-effectiveness of eight commercial DM programs. Other projects Nancy has led established Medicare's Chronic Care Data Warehouse that makes claims data available for clinical and health services researchers, longitudinal claims studies of disparities in beneficiary access to high-tech services, and Medicare's heart bypass global payment demonstration. Nancy also led teams in modifying Medicare physician and hospital prospective payment systems for public employees as well as Medicaid and Workers Compensation eligibles in West Virginia. It is obvious that she thrives on work- as long as it is intellectually rewarding and improves the human condition.

Technical Skills

To recap her technical skills, Nancy is a national expert on the following:

- Medicare physician and hospital payment systems and claims datasets
- Cardiovascular procedures and hospital responses to global payment methods
- Chronic disease models and implementation
- Quality of care process and outcome measures
- Hospital and physician organizational models

For example, Nancy was HCFA's expert consultant in creating analytic public use claims data sets, and how to make them as "user friendly" as possible. She used her extensive knowledge of heart disease acquired in Brigham & Women's Hospital to evaluate the outcomes and appropriateness of major heart surgeries performed by world famous surgeons in Medicare's "Centers of Excellence" Bypass Demonstration. Not an ivy-tower researcher, she interviewed many participating cardiac surgeons and cardiologists on their responses to global payment incentives to skimp on care. She then conducted qualitative and quantitative analyses of bypass mortality and morbidity controlling for numerous patient risk factors.

Quasi-experimental evaluation design and hierarchical sampling are second nature to her. One morning she may be designing a questionnaire for physicians and nurses, while in the afternoon she cleans data and conducts nonresponse bias tests and missing value imputations. She is comfortable running and interpreting ordinary least squares, logistic, Poisson count, and survival regression models. Theoretical, multiequation models do not intimidate her. She corrects other PhD researchers on their pairwise t-test calculations and knows when results are under powered. Her research integrity is unquestioned, which often gets her in trouble with government POs who have a preconceived notion of their program's success. Nancy studies very quickly and sees to the heart of a problem and any analytic challenge in short order. She is an excellent, efficient, technical, and policy writer and editor.

On many projects, Nancy's advanced clinical skills are often forgotten, not because they have atrophied, but because she functions more as a social scientist studying organizations, setting up research designs, and building and analyzing large claims data files. When called for, however, as on the evaluation of Medicare's new payment reductions for hospital-acquired conditions (HACs), Nancy leads cardiologists, internists, and nurses in the validation of hospital *International Classification of Diseases, Ninth Revision* (ICD-9; World Health Organization, 1977) coding and flaws in AHRQ's Patient Safety Indicator (PSI) algorithms. Her social science colleagues then see a "hidden" clinical side of her that reinforces her role with them as a scientific equal.

Leadership Style

Leaders can be "doers" or "motivators," but rarely both. Nancy would much prefer to lead staff through her own research: "Watch closely what, how, & how fast I do it." She has very high expectations of other researchers on her teams, high in terms of both work effort and quality of analysis. She does not "suffer fools gladly." I am not a psychologist, but her extraordinary intensity may be attributable to the fact she was a nurse in "another life" and feels that her colleagues should be quicker and better than she is given that their academic training was more focused on social science research than hers. I also believe that nurses (and physicians) are socially conditioned to work harder for more concentrated hours than most social scientists. They are trained to meet constant deadlines and get things done somehow, someway, under external orders and pressures.

However, Nancy cannot lead only by example. With three to ten researchers working for her on any project, she must delegate tasks and give direction. This challenges her because of her perfectionist personality and acute sensitivity to perceived failure at CMS when her team fails. She spreads herself thin across projects, mainly because she is so good technically and substantively across so many areas. Ultimately, Nancy must subordinate her absolute advantage to the iron law of comparative advantage and delegate extensively to other staff. Not surprisingly, having been exposed to a very high level of competence and internal work ethic while at the Brigham Hospital and Harvard, she sets a correspondingly high bar for all researchers working under her. Consequently, Nancy is not a mentor. She just does not have the time or the patience. She wants to successfully guide too many different programs, solve too many technical problems in health care cost and access to slow down and bring along another PhD or master's researcher "who shouldn't need mentoring anyway." How does she react to others' failures? Usually, Nancy gives staff a second chance then, if there is little improvement, she completes the task herself between 4:00 a.m. and 8:00 a.m., and finds a replacement.

Management

I distinguish pure management from research leadership styles. Some, like General Patton, are born to command armies in the field; others, like Eisenhower and Bradley, are more suited to manage entire combat theaters. Nancy is not a manager in the usual sense of the term. A good manager is one who motivates other managers, who recognizes the psychological needs and pressures faced by others. And most important, one who, if not totally accepting, is fairly tolerant of organizational bureaucracy. Her highly critical mind makes Nancy an outstanding leader of research but at the same time prevents her from being a great manager within a larger bureaucracy. No, Nancy is not a manager. She is a Chief Research Scientist—her title at RTI—a leader of researchers. It is a big difference.

Teaching

Nancy has worked her whole career either as a cardiac and oncology nurse or as a social science researcher. She has given many academic presentations on her research and has lectured on quality measurement in the University of Massachusetts' College of Nursing, but she has never taught full time in the classroom. Teaching leadership would best suit Nancy when lecturing occasionally to nurses and health service researchers on her many research projects. She has much to share, ranging from flaws in DM models to quality of care measures in hospitals to technical revisions in the Medicare fee schedule. She could also provide a unique perspective to PhD student nurses considering a nonacademic research career either in a private "think tank" or in a government agency.

Summary

What have I learned about research leadership from knowing Nancy? To be a successful researcher, especially in high-level, time-sensitive, projects, any nurse should

- love problem solving away from the patient's bedside,
- be able to abstract from the forest of minor complications to the "big picture,"
- have a burning drive to learn new analytic methods,
- have a strong work ethic,
- exhibit an almost fanatic attention to quantitative details, and
- communicate clearly and precisely in both the spoken and the written word.

Next, let me share some experiences I have had with nursing while working in government.

NURSES AT THE CENTERS FOR MEDICARE & MEDICAID SERVICES

With ever-rising health care costs that frustrate access to preventive and elective care, it is becoming increasingly important for nurses to play a role in health insurance and payment reforms. Nurses, traditionally, have been on the front lines managing urban and rural neighborhood health centers, on American Indian reservations, and fighting epidemics. They have been active in advocacy groups promoting research on crippling diseases and defending nurses' scope of practice in the workplace. But more often lately, they are taking up leadership positions in applied health services research in major health agencies. For example, nurses have been key in developing, refining, validating, and disseminating PSIs at the AHRQ in Washington. They have been on multidisciplinary teams conducting cost of illness and cost-effectiveness studies at the CDC in Atlanta. And rapidly growing roles for nurses can be found in the CMS. With an annual budget of nearly $800 billion, larger than the Pentagon's, CMS staff daily make decisions that directly affect 40 million elderly and disabled Medicare beneficiaries and 50 million Medicaid eligibles, and that affect several million physicians, nurses, hospitals, and other providers. Moreover, as private insurers increasingly follow Medicare's lead in payment policies, it is not a stretch to say that a few thousand Medicare/Medicaid staff, located in central offices in Baltimore, MD, and Washington, DC, have a major influence on 17% of all spending and employment in the entire country. Nurses fill key positions at CMS that make a difference, not in tens or hundreds of lives, but for millions and tens of millions of lives. They do so in myriad ways by affecting the way in which the Medicare and Medicaid programs pay for services, cover beneficiaries and services, and regulate providers.

Skills and Knowledge

What skills and knowledge are required of nurses to play these important roles? Naturally, they start with their unique clinical training, enhanced by their work experiences with individual patients in every kind of health care setting ranging from academic medical centers and nursing homes to home health agencies, physicians' offices, and remote health clinics. Working with economists, political scientists, sociologists, and lawyers at CMS, nurses bring a real-world perspective to the agency. But to be leaders at the higher echelons of policy, they need more. To lead at CMS, seeing "the big picture" is a necessity. Knowing how to manage a person's chronic diabetes is not enough. The nurse policy leader, for example, must also know the following:

- How to go about defining medical homes for reimbursement
- How to evaluate their effectiveness in managing a whole range of chronic diseases
- How to evaluate the evidence-based literature to debit hospital payment for HACs
- How to measure states' adherence to federal access regulations in their Medicaid programs

For this, they need a solid grounding in research design to discriminate valid from misleading research findings. They must develop, and have an appetite for, the arcane intricacies of the Medicare and Medicaid programs. Many academic researchers and leaders, including Congresspersons and most health care providers, eschew technical, "bureaucratic," knowledge. But just as nurses must know the bones and tissues of the human body in their role as caregivers, those playing a leadership role in setting national payment policy need to know the fundamental structure of the two largest health insurance programs in America, Medicare and Medicaid.

To play a true leadership role in payment policy, nurses need to have a working knowledge of statistics, behavioral economics, and medical sociology. Although knowing the difference between ordinary least squares and maximum likelihood regression is not essential, they are often called upon to review and interpret regression coefficients, logistic, survival, and Poisson count models, as well as tests of independent versus pairwise mean differences in payments and quality. Because so much of what they do involves financial calculations of demonstration success by actuaries, economists, and statisticians, and then generalizing from voluntary payment demonstrations to a national program, a basic grounding in health economics is invaluable. How do demand and supply factors come together in equilibrium to determine Medicare hospital admissions and readmissions? Why does excessive segmentation of the private insurance market by health status lead to the insurance "death spiral?" How should health improvements be measured in a physician gainsharing demonstration of hospital savings? And how can private supplemental insurance policies lead to unnecessary Medicare use? These are the kinds of questions that researchers ask and answer every day at CMS. But what, exactly, do nurses do in the largest public insurance program in the world?

CMS Nurse Leaders

As background, CMS is organized into two major divisions: (1) research and (2) operations. Currently, Marilyn Tavenner, RN, is the CMS Chief Administrator. She has overall responsibility for the entire agency. Renee Mentenech, RN, heads up the Office of Research & Evaluation at CMS. Her team of many PhD social scientists is primarily responsible for evaluating the many ongoing quality and pay for performance (P4P) demonstrations. Five other RNs currently work in her division, acting as POs. They solicit outside, independent, contract researchers and direct their evaluations of all internal and congressionally mandated demonstrations. Most concentrate on Medicare reforms, but a few are dedicated to reforms in the Medicaid program. Some nurses have doctorates in public health, one is a lawyer as well, and another has a PhD in epidemiology. Yet another RN is a lieutenant in the Public Health Service. Other nurses work throughout the research division—primarily in quality and access measurement. Consider two roles nurses play in setting and implementing health policy at CMS, one responsible for managing evaluations of P4P demonstrations and another measuring provider quality of care.

Demonstration Leadership

At any one time, CMS Office of Research has five to ten quality and payment demonstrations in various stages. Some will be getting started by negotiating participant terms and conditions, some will be in a lengthy data collection phase, and still others will be in the final report preparation stage for submission to the Congress. Medicare's High Cost Beneficiary Demonstration is a good example. Lorraine Johnson, RN, is heading up the evaluation in the Office of Research, having replaced David Bott, who is now the editor in chief of the *Health Care Financing Review*. This demonstration tests provider-based DM interventions at Texas Tech Medical

Center, Montefiore Hospital in New York, Massachusetts General Hospital, and elsewhere. Providers are paid upfront monthly fees for managing their patients with high medical costs. As the researcher in charge of the evaluation, Lorraine would produce the Request for Proposals (RFP) that solicit external evaluators of the demonstration. The RFP describes the problem with chronic, high-cost, Medicare beneficiaries, lists many research questions to be answered, explains the financial and quality terms and conditions in participant contracts, suggests possible research designs, control groups, and statistical approaches, and provides a schedule of deliverables. The RFP author is also responsible for developing estimates of evaluation costs to guide research organizations bidding on the contract. The PO usually chairs the internal group selecting the evaluation contractor, in this case RTI, using strict federal guidelines.

Once in place, the evaluation team meets with the CMS PO and produces a final evaluation design. The PO personally critiques the design and solicits comments from his or her colleagues in both the research and demonstrations groups. As the evaluation proceeds, Lorraine reviews and comments on interim findings and might accompany the evaluation team on site visits. She arranges for CMS data use agreements that permit access by the outside evaluation team to the millions of confidential Medicare Part A and B claims that are necessary to evaluate intervention utilization, quality, and cost savings. Lorraine is responsible for reviewing and commenting on the scientific rigor and objectivity of each report—usually about 100 pages each. These reports involve complex quasi-experimental research designs with sophisticated nonparametric and parametric regression methods. They also include qualitative critiques of how DM was implemented based on site visits. Her leadership was tested in the phrasing of report conclusions that are often not favorable to participants. Several DM organizations contested some of RTI's findings and asked for major revisions. Lorraine, in conjunction with RTI staff, must decide on which edits to make without compromising the scientific import of the findings. On other demonstrations, CMS's POs have had to respond to Senators John Kerry and Ted Kennedy's queries, motivated by participant dissatisfaction with the findings, about the independence and rigor of the evaluation. CMS POs, as the federal point persons, quickly learn how to deal, sensitively, with criticisms from participants, Congress, and occasionally, White House staff. Once a report is accepted, Lorraine will make it available on the CMS website and share it with Congress. She will also contribute her knowledge of the demonstration's success and challenges at future CMS staff meetings tasked with implementing the new Affordable Care Act (ACA) passed by the Congress in 2010.

Quality of Care

Nurses in other divisions at CMS are leaders and parts of teams dealing with the quality of care that beneficiaries receive. Three examples highlight the critical role nurses play in this field. First, CMS staff must address provider workforce issues through their regulatory authority. The most contentious regulations have to do with allowing nonphysicians to bill Part B of Medicare directly, thereby encroaching on the previously unique privilege accorded physicians. Direct billing is a necessary condition for practice independence, nowhere more contentious than in the delivery of anesthesia. Although the majority of anesthetics were delivered by certified registered nurse anesthetists (CRNAs) in the early years of Medicare, CRNAs were not granted direct billing until 1988. The American Society of Anesthesiologists (ASA) fought this decision, and still does, primarily on the grounds of poor outcomes without anesthesiologist supervision. Nurses and physicians at CMS are frequently called upon to adjudicate complaints by the ASA. In 2001, for example, they conducted a thorough review of the literature on patient safety and found no compelling evidence of any difference in surgical outcomes related to anesthesia provider. Consequently, CMS rescinded the requirement that CRNAs must be supervised by the surgeon if an anesthesiologist is not on the case. Similar workforce payment decisions have been (and likely will be) made for midwives, nurse practitioners, and other nurse professionals to address the high cost of health care and growing shortage of primary care physicians—especially in rural areas. It is critical that well-trained nurses play an active role within CMS as these decisions are made. However, leadership will require a thorough understanding of medicine, how to conduct a critical literature review, and how to collaborate with physicians in setting national policy.

In a second example, the 2006 Deficit Reduction Act (DRA) authorized CMS to begin to penalize hospitals financially for complications, or what are now termed HACs. Ten conditions were identified by CMS clinicians ranging from falls to surgical and catheter infections to pressure ulcers. Many of the 10 could be considered negligent nursing care. (It was puzzling that physicians were not financially penalized for any HACs, including air embolisms, foreign bodies left in after surgery, or mediastinitis.) Nurses work on CMS teams deciding which complications to raise to the level of an HAC, and interacting with clinicians at AHRQ who originally developed the PSI software used to identify HACs. They reviewed the clinical literature on evidence-based guidelines that justified an "avoidable" complication. Often, the literature is not specific enough and nurses and physicians at CMS had to judge whether the HAC software was sensitive and specific enough not to unjustly penalize hospitals. Next, they decided how much to penalize hospitals using the complex DRG (diagnosis-related group) payment algorithms and taking the degree of a hospital's responsibility for the HAC into consideration. Then they developed new HAC candidates for consideration as requested by Congress. Finally, they are overseeing the evaluation of payment reductions in HAC rates and any unintended consequences (e.g., discharging patients earlier, failing to code complications).

Yet a third example comes from Medicare's many DM demonstrations in which participants must maintain or improve quality to keep their management fees. Nurses and physicians needed to establish process-of-care markers for heart failure and diabetics in randomized trials. These included such measures as beta blocker and blood pressure testing for heart failure and lipid tests for diabetics. Because DM groups were allowed to suggest their own markers, clinicians had to evaluate their appropriateness and determine how much of the management fees would be put at risk for quality lapses. Nurses in the quality group at CMS also draw upon their advanced clinical training to set up Medicare's Hospital Compare website for patients, evaluate new cardiovascular diagnostic and treatment interventions, and initiate numerous other value-based purchasing initiatives legislated under the ACA.

How can nurses prepare for a career in setting state and national health policy? The answer is to invest in a PhD in health services research.

PhD NURSING STUDENTS

I have now taught four cohorts of nurses in the PhD program in the University of Massachusetts Boston's College of Nursing. They enter with a broad mix of experience, some with master's degrees, others on a fast track with just bachelor of arts or bachelor of science degrees. A few have been senior nurse managers in prestigious hospitals and cancer clinics or managed neighborhood health clinics. Others work for health departments, nursing associations, or on nursing units in Boston hospitals while in school. Several were born and received their initial nurse training in Armenia, Pakistan, India, Kenya, Puerto Rico, and Taiwan. All have decided to leave bedside nursing to make a change in the system.

The graduate curriculum is focused on health policy and population health research. The few who returned to senior nurse manager positions with their PhDs take advantage of their access to patients to lead NIH-funded grant research. Their PhD degrees provide an entrée to clinical societies, international conferences, and NIH grant review sections at the regional and national levels. Other nurses use their advanced degrees to develop and implement new health policies at the state and national levels. To do so requires a broader and deeper knowledge of economic and political theories, medical sociology, and advanced research methods than one gets with a clinically focused nursing education, or DNP.

To fulfill leadership roles as researchers, students receive core courses in policy formulation and implementation, health economics and finance, basic statistics and multivariate regression, research methods, and secondary data analysis. Other courses introduce students to health disparities, qualitative methods, population health and epidemiology, and how to conduct integrated literature reviews. Prior to taking their comprehensive examination, students are placed in a state legislator's office or public health agency for an in-depth internship to learn the practical requirements of developing and enacting new health policies. By the end of their coursework, students should be able to converse and work collaboratively as equals with other social scientists—economists, political scientists, sociologists, and epidemiologists. They should also be able to design and execute research studies that involve complex multivariate analysis. Many learn a statistical language (e.g., SAS®; IBM SPSS; Stata®) well enough to conduct their own quantitative analyses. Others prefer qualitative analyses of organization and system change but still are capable of directing and interpreting statistical analyses of program impacts (e.g., mandatory nurse staffing ratios). Although after graduation none of the students have become health economists, political theorists, or epidemiologists, they have learned enough theory and methods from the other disciplines to leverage the value added of their previous clinical training in setting national health policy. Let me share three examples of students who embarked on a research career.

After passing her comprehensive examination, Terry Eng Kahlert is currently working part time at RTI while completing her PhD. Her PhD schoolwork, coupled with her longtime interest in hospital complications, prepared her well to collaborate with the RTI team of cardiologists and health service researchers in evaluating Medicare's HAC payment penalty program. Terry critically reviewed the evidence-based guidelines literature supporting federal expansion of the initial ten HACs. She has also been interviewing policy makers in other states regarding their implementation of HAC financial penalties and the challenges they have faced in implementing the new rules. Her thesis builds on her evaluation research using a combination of qualitative hospital interviews and multivariate modeling of hospital characteristics explaining their responses to financial penalties. Terry's research training is perfectly suited to a career in state or national health policy design and implementation.

Rebecca Penders is beginning her journey in secondary data analysis by analyzing CDC's Infant Feeding Practices Survey. It is a very complex, multiwave survey that captures detailed information on breastfeeding activities over a 12-month postnatal period. She is estimating a two-stage model, first, to explain why 477 of 3,030 new mothers decided not to breastfeed at all, and second, what economic, cultural, employment, and family variables curtail the recommended 12 months of breastfeeding of new infants. She is becoming proficient in using Stata® logistic and Cox proportional hazard software to isolate the marginal effects of each variable on breastfeeding behaviors. When Rebecca is done, she will be ready to lead new quantitative research on her own in a field in which most nurses have traditionally been limited to qualitative analyses.

Mercy Kamau, like Rebecca, is learning how to conduct quantitative analyses using secondary data. Mercy's interest is cardiovascular disease, an interest sparked by the College of Nursing's innovative heart disease prevention program in low-income Boston neighborhoods. But like most foreign-trained nurses, Mercy also wanted to study the spread of the disease in Kenya, her own country. Always enterprising, Mercy discovered a comprehensive survey by the World Health Organization (WHO) of health behaviors in 17 developing countries, including Kenya. Although implemented under rigorous oversight by WHO staff, the survey presents many more data challenges than U.S.-focused surveys like Rebecca's. For example, practically no respondent in Kenya reportedly was diagnosed with angina, but Mercy was certain that the problem was widespread and underreported because of the usual international focus on infectious diseases. Searching the voluminous database, Mercy found another question that asked whether the person had been having chest pains. She is analyzing responses to this question using multivariate regression based on lifestyle habits (e.g., poor nutrition, smoking), education, occupation, and tribal differences. When she completes her research, she will have the statistical and epidemiological background to be a leader in international health research in her own country and elsewhere in Africa. Mercy's rare combination of clinical training, research training, and native Kenyan background provides a springboard to leadership in a field dearly lacking in indigenous talent and research training.

CONCLUSION

There are over 2 million nurses in the United States today (BLS Statistics, in U.S. Census Statistical Abstract of the U.S., 2001). In the last 30 years, the number of nurses has tripled as the demand for health care services has exploded. Nursing is by far the largest well-paying career for women, a fact that has encouraged more men to enter the field. Nursing is becoming increasingly professionalized, as evidenced by the new requirement for advanced practice nurses to obtain a doctorate in nursing practice. For those who wish to make a change in the system, however, a sound research background is required, not only in advanced clinical fields such as pharmacology, but in several social sciences as well. Physicians, too, continue to enter policy research in increasing numbers and play dominant roles in key public health agencies. The current head of CMS is a physician and, naturally, so is the head of the NIH. But nurses, too, are playing more prominent decision-making roles in key agencies. A nurse is now second in command at CMS. Another is head of the Office of Research at CMS.

But if more nurses are going to be leaders in formulation of health policies, especially regarding finances, they will need to overcome their aversion to mathematics, statistics, and complex social modeling. Accomplishing this is easier said than done. Most have been socialized on the job to play a subordinate role following orders with little encouragement of creative thinking. If nurses want to play on the same field as physicians in the highly technical world of policy making, they must substantially upgrade their technical skills. They must embrace the languages and thought processes of quantitative research. When a physician mistakenly interprets a logistic odds ratio in a meeting, they must correct him. When a Congressman draws a wrong inference from a survival hazard function, a nurse should be there to correct him. Knowledge is power, and technical knowledge in today's world approaches absolute power. Policy makers, in the end, must defer to those with the best science. And in an ideal world, policy makers would be accomplished researchers in an earlier life. For nurses to publish in the *Journal of the American Medical Association* and the *New England Journal of Medicine*, for nurses to run CMS and the Department of Health & Human Services, for nurses to actually *prove* that a new health program works or not, they need to accept the challenge of learning something really hard, really different; to wit, they need to acquire the tools of the research trade. If they do, like Nancy McCall, they will be invaluable contributors to the future health of people everywhere.

REFERENCE

World Health Organization. (1997). *International classification of diseases, ninth revision*. Geneva, Switzerland: Author.

8

The Essence of Excellent Health Care Delivery

Michael J. Dowling

Commentary
by Joyce J. Fitzpatrick

A *ccording to Dowling, leaders promote change; this is accomplished by understanding the present, selectively forgetting the past, and creating a brighter future. Leaders understand the way things have been done and know that there is a better way to the future. Importantly, they can articulate their vision of the future for others.*

Nurse leaders and aspiring nurse leaders could learn the important lesson that Dowling learned at an early age from his mother: "Never let your situation limit your potential." Although as nurse leaders we often find ourselves sitting at an uneven table, marginalized by gender and profession, like Dowling, we can create our preferred future. Another important lesson from Dowling is the advice that strong leaders MUST draw apostles who are riveted by the leader's vision. We need more riveting leaders in nursing now at a time when health care needs more leaders.

Dowling describes the opportunities for leadership and the essential ingredients for excellence in health care delivery. He considers one of the key ingredients the "right people" and believes that nurses can be the catalysts to lead the health care team. Although those of us in nursing often talk about nurses as catalysts for change, we have not framed the message in the precise language of Dowling, that is, catalysts to lead. Dowling also supports a culture of learning to create nurse leaders, and importantly, argues for breaking down the silos in health care education and delivery. Within the large health care system he leads, he has placed nurses in key strategic roles, not only to elevate the profession, but also to improve patient care.

Key focus areas: strategic vision, catalyst, interprofessional, forward-thinker, change

My mother was a great inspiration to me on my journey to lead an almost $6 billion health care network—the largest in New York State, employing more than 10,000 nurses. Deaf from an early age, my mother had very little formal education. She was a voracious reader, however. Her motto was never let your situation limit your potential. I took that to heart coming from modest family circumstances.

A midwife delivered me in a country farmhouse in the south of Ireland, and I grew up working on local farms, milking cows and doing other chores. My home had a thatched roof and a dirt floor, but I remember us reading Shakespeare by candlelight. My father was disabled from arthritis so I became familiar and interested in health and human services at a young age. My modest beginnings instilled in me a thirst for knowledge, a fervor to create a better life, and a strong desire to make a difference in the health and human services arena.

I left home at a young age, working in steel mills in England to support my family. I was 17 when I came to New York, where I got a job working in the electrical room of a Circle Line ship. The first in my family to attend college, I earned my bachelor's degree from Ireland's University College Cork in 1971, working part time as a construction worker, longshoreman, and plumber. I also used a series of blue-collar jobs to help fund my master's degree from Fordham University in 1973. Before joining North Shore-Long Island Jewish (LIJ) Health System in 1995, I worked briefly for Empire Blue Cross/Blue Shield, served in New York State government for 12 years as the health and human services advisor to then-Governor Mario Cuomo, and was a member of the faculty and administration at Fordham.

I continue teaching at Harvard and at North Shore-LIJ Health System's corporate university, the Center for Learning and Innovation (CLI), and serving on many health care boards. My commitment to health care has apparently inspired the careers of both of my children, although I did not deliberately encourage them in this direction. My son works in radiology, and my daughter graduated from nursing school and plans to dedicate herself to caring for patients with cancer. Her commitment and performance in her rigorous studies give me confidence that she will make a mark in her special calling.

CHANGE AGENTS AND CATALYSTS

My upbringing and my drive to create a better future for my family and me shaped my definition of leadership. Leadership is all about promoting change. Effective leaders understand present conditions, try to selectively forget the past, and create a brighter future. I have been described as having "a relentless attention to management" to create one of the best health systems in the United States, but I distinguish leadership from management. Management is doing what you now do very well—meeting deadlines, hitting targets, and putting processes in place to get things done. Sometimes managers are very good leaders, but not always. It is not automatic. We need both managers and leaders in a health system as large as North Shore-LIJ, but leaders are critical for taking us to the next level. Leaders understand the way things have always been done, know that there is a better way to improve the situation and can articulate their vision of the future to others. Having a mother who was hearing impaired taught me that you have to be very creative about how you communicate. My mother would read lips, but none of us in the family knew sign language. We were able to communicate with my mother, however, because we learned to adapt well, to be creative in getting attention, and to simplify concepts to convey our ideas.

Describing the future and helping others envision the future of health care is more important today than ever before because of the pressing clinical and financial demands on the industry. In many ways, we are suffering due to our success in health care in improving longevity and the quality of life. Because more people are living longer and straining their finances to cover their health care-related expenses, it is more imperative than ever for leaders to demonstrate how to deliver quality health care more cost-effectively. Strong leaders must draw apostles to them, not because they *have* to follow, but because they are riveted by their vision of what the future should look like and are engaged in the cause. Leadership is not about titles or positions. Martin Luther King Jr., for example, did not have a formal organizational title, but he inspired millions with his dream for human rights and social equity. Leadership is about influencing others to do the right thing and not mistaking means for end results.

EMPLOYING TOOLS EFFECTIVELY

My good friend and authority on the topic of leadership, Jim Champy, advocates that to reengineer our current health care system will take widespread use of information technology (IT) to eliminate inefficient practices. Like me, however, he knows that IT is merely a tool for sharing data more freely, coordinating care better, and improving clinical outcomes. Informatics will continue to play a large part in health care, including in the role of nursing, but you can have the best technology in the world and it would not work without the right people.

The bulk of health care today and in the future will be spent on people who are older. Thanks to the new health care reform law, more than 30 million insured people are entering the health care system as our population continues to age—82 million people during the next decade will turn 65. It takes a whole team to care for patients—nurses, doctors, social workers, rehabilitation specialists, dietitians, among others—but nurses can be the catalyst to lead the team and ensure that it works effectively.

North Shore-LIJ Health System is the nation's second-largest, nonprofit secular health system with 15 hospitals that contain more than 5,600 beds and a total workforce of more than 43,000 employees. Because of the strength of their numbers—almost one quarter of our workforce—and their unique education and capabilities, nurses are key leaders in our health system. They are the essence of a health care delivery system. Nurses serve as executive directors of several of North Shore-LIJ's hospitals, including Forest Hills Hospital in northern Queens, North Shore University Hospital in Manhasset, and Southside Hospital in Bay Shore. A nurse is also regional executive director with responsibility over several North Shore-LIJ hospitals. Nurses, as most of us know, spend more time than anyone else with the patient or customer, including in acute care, subacute care, psychiatric care, long-term care, home health, and hospice and community health. Astute physicians know the value of depending on good nurses and making them equal partners in patient care.

CULTURE OF LEARNING

To make North Shore-LIJ one of the best health systems in the United States, offering the highest quality of care and financial success, I have sought to build a consistent corporate-learning culture in which nurses play an integral role. One of my first actions when I became CEO in 2002 was to create the CLI, symbolizing my commitment to lifelong learning and inviting leaders to regularly engage their staff in educational programs. Health care leaders visit from across the country to observe our corporate university, including the Cleveland Clinic, one of the largest private medical centers in the world.

    I felt so strongly about the contribution of nursing to leadership that I tapped a nurse, Kathleen Gallo, RN, PhD, MBA, to be Chief Learning Officer and lead the Center, reporting directly to me.

    Our CLI promotes a culture dedicated to excellence, innovation, teamwork, and continuous change. Through learning opportunities, employees develop the knowledge, attitude, and skills that support the North Shore-LIJ Health System's business goals. As Senior Vice President and Chief Learning Officer, Kathy is responsible for CLI, as well as for our Patient Safety Institute (PSI), one of the largest multidisciplinary clinical simulation centers in the country. A nurse also directs all daily educational activities at the PSI. Kathy's responsibilities include the development and implementation of the organizational learning strategy to support the health system's business imperatives and the advancement of human resources to a strategic business partner for the health system.

With more than 25 years of leadership in emergency services, Kathy has also written articles on trauma, nursing research, interprofessional education, and leadership development in nursing. She speaks regularly on such topics as creating a world-class learning organization, building performance teams, leadership development, the role of the professional doctorate, and patient safety.

MODEL FOR NURSING PRACTICE

In addition to North Shore-LIJ's corporate university, which continues to be the largest in the health care industry, I created an Institute for Nursing in 2004. The goal is to promote quality patient care through the advancement of nursing science at every level of practice by integrating nursing research, education, professional growth, and outcome studies. The Institute, led by Senior Vice President and Chief Nurse Executive Maureen White, RN, empowers our 10,000+ nurses to share and enhance their knowledge, expertise, and potential within a supportive and focused environment. It melds nursing practice, research, and education to facilitate a system-wide standard of care and set a national model for nursing practice. As chief nurse executive and director of our Institute for Nursing, Maureen's overarching goal is to create a healthy work environment and develop future nursing leaders within the health system.

To support the culture advocated by the Institute for Nursing, it is worth noting that North Shore-LIJ contributes more than $2 million a year in tuition reimbursement to more than 1,000 nurses in any given year who are seeking advanced degrees at one of 15 colleges and universities nationwide with whom North Shore-LIJ has developed nursing school affiliations. In 2006, for instance, North Shore-LIJ developed a custom-tailored doctorate of nursing practice (DNP) program with Case Western Reserve University's Frances Payne Bolton School of Nursing in Cleveland, Ohio. North Shore-LIJ has financed all tuition costs for 64 of its nurses in varying disciplines, recognizing the value of investing in future leaders in nursing practice, clinical research, and business administration. More than 125 nonnurses at North Shore-LIJ have also earned associate's degrees in nursing.

Among the factors behind the health system's focus on nursing education is research showing a significant correlation between higher levels of nursing education and improved quality outcomes, lower mortality, and fewer adverse events. With input from Maureen, North Shore-LIJ developed a policy that now requires all new nurses to have a bachelor of nursing science (BSN) degree or earn one within 5 years. Nurses already on staff who have not earned their BSN are strongly encouraged to continue their education and take advantage of the health system's tuition reimbursement program.

Maureen's instincts and guidance have been invaluable to me personally and to the entire organization. She has held numerous leadership positions at our hospitals and has been the chief nurse executive since the 1997 merger of North Shore Hospital System and LIJ Medical Center in 1997 that formed the North Shore-LIJ Health System.

Both Maureen and Kathy have the broad, strategic vision critical for advancing learning across our massive health care system and beyond and have hands-on knowledge of the art and science of nursing. Both nursing leaders have a firm grasp of the overall health care landscape, are not hostage to precedent, and are not only willing, but eager to change the status quo because they know the biggest risk taken to create a successful future is not taking *any* risk. Kathy and Maureen understand the high-level trends occurring in health care today—value-based reimbursement, complete transparency, and promoting care across the whole continuum—and have the credibility and trust of others to effect change.

Their strategic direction has led to the creation of many new programs and plans for the future. A new system-wide interprofessional orientation program, for instance, incorporates registered nurses, nurse practitioners, and physician assistants to foster collaboration and teamwork and promote quality and safety for our patients.

Breaking Down Silos

Nurses at North Shore-LIJ Health System are not educated in a silo. They are systematically engaged in learning with clinicians from other disciplines to bring a holistic perspective to patient care. This multidisciplinary approach to learning is one of the primary reasons for the development of the PSI. We sponsor two leadership retreats—summer and winter—that are structured to bring together nurses with physicians and clinical and administrative leaders and expose them to the broader goals and mission of the health system. I also encourage nurses to take advantage of informal opportunities to network and socialize with physicians. The greater the communication between nurses and doctors and the more they understand each other's challenges and issues, the more we can improve patient care. Health care delivery is a team sport and nurses make natural captains because of their ability to work so effectively in an interdisciplinary fashion to bridge the silo mentality.

DEVELOPING FACULTY

North Shore-LIJ Health System continues to evolve to meet the needs of the community. Because facilities shape how clinicians deliver health care, nurses are very involved in helping us design such facilities as the Katz Women's Hospital at Long Island Jewish Hospital in New Hyde Park and North Shore University Hospital. Nurses are also integrally involved in helping us create the curriculum for a new master's-level school of nursing, which we plan to introduce in a couple of years. There may be a shortage of nurses, but we have no shortage of people who want to become nurses. That is a big difference. The reason there may be a shortage of nurses is that many nursing schools are not equipped to accommodate all the qualified candidates.

There are two options when facing a problem—you can admire the problem or you can do something to solve it. We are not sitting back complaining about the lack of nursing faculty. We are developing our own by educating our nurses to become organizational leaders. Because the demands of the future will require more holistic services, our plan is to have the nurses we teach participate in classes with students who attend our new medical school (the Hofstra North Shore-LIJ School of Medicine), which opened in August 2011.

Placing nurses in key strategic roles at North Shore-LIJ Health System is elevating the status and knowledge base of nursing and improving care for patients. My mother would have been gratified to see me in a position to hire women in leadership and to make a difference in health and human services. She would have been especially pleased to see her granddaughter dedicate herself to nursing—one of the most trusted professions yesterday, today, and tomorrow.

9

Hiring as a Pathway to Understanding Leadership

Karen Gross

Commentary
by Joyce J. Fitzpatrick

*A*s a college president, Gross has been confronted with many leadership challenges. To illustrate qualities of nurse leaders, she relates the story of lessons learned when hiring a new nurse leader for the academic unit at a small, rural, private liberal arts and sciences college. She learned of the existing nurse leader network, individuals tightly linked by their commitment to the profession and to developing future generations of nurse leaders. These nurse leaders demonstrated the transferability of their caring nursing skills and willingness to help others achieve goals and advance the profession.

Gross also describes the importance of learning "silo busting" in any leadership role, a skill not easily practiced within the silo-rich academic communities. Yet interdisciplinary interaction is an important leadership skill that will benefit leaders of all disciplines, and students need to see this model within the learning environment. Gross further describes the importance of empowering all individuals to think of themselves as leaders, rather than embracing the hierarchical positional leadership model that often dominates our institutions. Accordingly, we need to communicate in bold and creative ways that you

> *can lead every minute of every day if you seize the opportunities.*
>
> *Gross expects the nursing faculty and students on her campus to become leaders in crossing the disciplinary divide, and she is creating opportunities to ensure their success. She believes that we owe it to our students to invest in their development from the beginning of their education, so that they also learn to connect with each other, create the important networks, and transport their caring skills into the leadership arenas.*

Key focus areas: visionary, mentor, communication, risk-taker, "silo busting"

Reflecting on leadership occurs at many junctures and in many contexts in the life of a college president. Most recently, we were searching for a new chair of our nursing division (something equivalent to a dean position at our institution). That search—now successfully concluded—gave me an opportunity to reflect on what type of health care leader we were seeking at Southern Vermont College (SVC), the small, rural, private, career-launching liberal arts and sciences institution I lead. But the process enabled much more than that.

Although not a health care professional, I spent more than 15 months thinking about leadership in the context of nursing. The whole search process—from creating the job description to identifying a quality candidates' pool to interviewing and ultimately selecting a divisional chair to helping the successful candidate see the fit with our institution—allowed me to consider what qualities are critical to nursing leadership within the academy. And it allowed me to consider whether the qualities of a leader in nursing were different from the qualities needed by all leaders within and outside higher education.

Beyond that, and of perhaps equal if not greater value, searching for a nursing divisional chair created opportunities for me to reflect on several other key questions within the SVC sphere such as how can we engender leadership qualities among our nursing graduates? And importantly, how do the lessons learned from this nursing leadership search transport themselves in other fields across the college?

In this broader thought exercise, I was regularly thinking about strategies for enabling our graduates across the institution to grow within their professions over the coming decades. In a challenge confronting all leaders today, I pondered what measureable competencies we are engendering and aspiring to engender in our graduates.

I begin this chapter by describing the key lessons learned about nursing leadership within the academy and then share how those lessons unfolded in practice. I appreciate that this is the inverse of how many articles normally proceed; usually, the stories are first and the lessons culled from them appear later. But, in this instance, I think the lessons learned help animate the story. Then, I reflect on how these lessons learned provide some insight into strategies for training the next generation of nursing leaders.

In brief, this chapter reflects lessons about leadership that occurred not from leading per se but from the process of hiring an academic nursing leader.

EIGHT LESSONS LEARNED

Here are the key lessons learned:

One: There is a shortage of nurses to lead within the academy, and part of the reason, I suspect, is that we were and continue to be too slow to move nurses into leadership positions (in part because we define leadership too narrowly and hierarchically). This resulting shortage threatens our capacity to grow quality nursing programs, which in turn constrains workforce development.

Two: The "conventional" search processes for finding a nursing leader are not optimal (at least within a small, rural institution). Also, try as we did to get the job description right, it did not do the job of animating our needs. Instead, institutions need to adopt out-of-the-box approaches, in this case ones that involved the institution's president. These approaches, although beneficial on several levels, take time. This means a protracted search process is inevitable.

Three: The existing leaders within the nursing profession are tightly connected with each other and more than willing, once aware of the needs, to assist in identifying leadership candidates, without being competitive or threatened. The networks among existing nursing leaders signaled the commitment of their profession to caring for its own and to developing leadership capacity in the next generation.

Four: The skills needed to lead a nursing program within a college or university extend far beyond the ever-so-important "traditional" health care competencies. Nursing leaders of the future, including those within the academy, need a wide range of skills such as proficiency in their field; appreciation for both the art and science of nursing; extraordinary communication capacities to a range of constituencies; calmness in the face of crises; financial acumen; creativity; a willingness to innovate and take risks; and a respect for disciplines apart from their own.

Five: A successful nursing leader within academia does not need to come from a single, preordained pathway (i.e., from a faculty or a chair position) but can come with transportable leadership skill sets developed in other health care settings such as hospitals, nursing homes, or research facilities.

Six: Within the academy, we need to do more—and as a college president, I need to do more—to encourage "silo-crossing." We need to message about interdisciplinary interaction and its importance, including, for example, raising monies to enable coteaching, encouraging panels that bring the disciplines together, and rewarding (with money or other accolades) those who see the merits of this approach.

Seven: We have an opportunity, which we do not leverage sufficiently, to facilitate ways for our nursing students, including those at different stages of their academic progression, to work together even more effectively, reducing the competition among them and enabling caring not just for their patients but for each other.

Eight: Within the academy, we need to find ways to encourage leadership skills among our faculty and students. We tend to view leadership as hierarchical but as this search suggested, leaders do not need to come up the traditional route to be successful if we are bold and creative in how we assess leadership skills. Moreover, there are opportunities to lead every minute of every day from, as Chief Executive Officer Terri Ludwig phrases it, "your seat." Building leadership capacity early and often in our health care students and faculty is key, and we need to be deliberate about facilitating leadership development within our community.

These lessons are extrapolations based on our just-completed search process; indeed, had the search been shorter or more traditional, my learning would have been shortchanged. With the benefit of 20/20 hindsight, our search was more revelatory than I expected.

SEARCHING FOR A NURSING LEADER

We began the search process, as is common in many institutions within and outside higher education, with crafting a job description. That sounds easy enough but not all descriptions are alike, and one can use a description to provide a very clear signal as to what one is looking for among successful candidates. What is also clear is that the description is often an unintentional or unconscious response to shortcomings or strengths (or both) in the leader who previously held the position for which one is now searching. The latter realization might account for why the styles of leadership within an institution often swing like a pendulum as we are prone to hiring in response to past experience rather than focusing on what new skills are needed in a new leader so that person can move a program forward.

Beyond the usual experiences and professional acumen within the field of nursing, we knew that we were seeking a leader who could grow our program, expanding our offerings not just in numbers but also in approaches to teaching and learning. We wanted someone who could be innovative within a regulated industry. We wanted someone who would work well as part of a college-wide Divisional Council, a group that brings together leaders across disciplines within the institution. And, we knew from our nursing accreditors that we needed a candidate with a terminal degree: a PhD or a DNP.

As hard as we worked on the job description that we posted, it did not quite capture the leader I thought our institution needed— a rare combination of a person with organizational talent, creative thinking, interpersonal communication strengths across an array of constituencies from students to their parents to faculty within and outside the nursing field, to accreditors to local and regional medical facilities, among others. We were also seeking someone with the capacity to work ably across silos.

Let me explain this latter point, which is, for me, a central tenet of what is needed in today's nursing leaders.

We are a career-launching college with a liberal arts and sciences core; as such, although we train nurses, we see ourselves as training thoughtful individuals across a range of professions. Indeed, all of our students—regardless of their major—take virtually the same required core courses and these interdisciplinary offerings matter. These courses are what help us ensure that we are training individuals with the capacity to problem solve, to think deeply about issues, to ask questions, to ponder links across fields that are seemingly disparate, to give back to their communities in meaningful ways, and to engage in our democratic process.

It is for this reason that we wanted a nursing leader who could do more than lead our nursing faculty in creating licensed nurses, as important as that is. We wanted a leader who could help our nursing faculty become leaders on our campus and help our students realize their broader leadership capacities. This is not an easy request. It requires skill sets often not measured effectively in searches.

Initially, we launched a search in the manner most common in higher education: advertising in appropriate publications where prospective chairs/deans might look, listing the position on our own website, sending and placing flyers in schools with graduate schools of nursing, and investigating the hiring of a search firm to provide us with assistance. From our head of Human Resources to our provost to our interim head of nursing, we tried to outreach to schools of nursing with graduate programs and to people we knew. To make a long story short, these traditional avenues did not work. We had few job applicants, and those who applied did not seem to meet the needed qualifications. Search firms, when candid, expressed a lack of interest in our search: the chair salary was too low, the pool of candidates they served was unlikely to resettle in Vermont, and the firm fee was too high for a small institution like ours to justify.

In short order, we realized that the conventional approach to searching for academic chairs was not going to work. I realized that if we were going to find a chair within some reasonable time frame, we had to search differently. We had to work through less formal channels and tap into the larger networks that nurse leaders, particularly those in academia, maintain. In short, I personally needed to get to know many nurses in positions of leadership within nursing schools. To gain access to this group, I was fortunate in that the president of a neighboring college had previously been a provost at an institution with a large and very successful nursing division and the president's wife had a doctoral degree in nursing and had come to our campus to speak to our community on several occasions. Through these two individuals, I was able to connect with some remarkable leaders within nursing education (and in the interest of full disclosure, two of them are the editors of this book).

I met and talked with a host of nursing leaders frequently over a period of months. They in turn introduced me to other leaders in nursing, and I even made a "pitch" to a meeting of nursing educators in Massachusetts. I shared with everyone with whom I spoke what we were searching for and why. I explained the kind of leader we were seeking; they asked good questions. They were consummate professionals. One of them visited our campus to help us. Another of them assisted us in finding a curriculum consultant. To stay au courant, I read about nursing education; I visited our simulation lab frequently; I had Benner's books on my nightstand; I spoke to the chief nursing officer of our local hospital; I spent time with our interim nursing chair reflecting on our program.

In this process, I became clearer about my view that nursing leaders needed to cross the disciplinary divide, and I shared with anyone who would listen a small subset of examples of what we were doing at SVC. For example, I spoke with nursing leaders I met about our first-year course in which a wide range of SVC students studied their own DNA to discover their roots, a course that involves a range of disciplines (science, history, geography, art) and culminates in mounting an exhibit in a local museum. I shared a pilot anatomy and physiology course that provided a professional health care tutor (who was an SVC nursing graduate), used physicians to teach segments of the course, created an avatar patient (replete with a chart) who exhibited every disease imaginable and stayed with students throughout the year, and deployed audience response technology to reinforce learning. It was these stories—the tales of what we were doing—that enabled those helping me identify candidates; paper job descriptions were not the coin of the realm—describing in-the-trenches opportunities to innovate were.

As I shared these examples, current and prospective courses flooded my mind: the use of art to inform observational skills among our health care, criminal justice, and psychology students through the use of a painting/print collection donated to the college; a joint nursing/criminal justice course in which one of our simulation patients is a crime victim, and our nursing students and criminal justice students would work together starting with an initial encounter in an emergency department and ending with testifying in a courtroom; a neuropsychology course that addressed Alzheimer's disease and included review of actual case files and an opportunity to visit a local research facility dedicated to investigating solutions to memory loss; and a summer research course involving research on telomere length in patients with dementia. I became fixated with finding a leader who could see the value in cross-disciplinary education for nursing students. I spoke about these courses on campus. I got the Sim boy to speak with the aid of a faculty member, and for months, I had him sitting in my office greeting visitors as I shared the value of hands-on, patient-sensitive learning that crossed the disciplines. Sim boy met prospective health care students but also criminal justice students and psychology students.

Here's what the nursing educators I encountered did: They listened and they heard and they connected with their colleagues and their former students and their friends. Remarkable.

It is because of and through the network of nurses in academia that we identified possible candidates for our chair position. What I learned through this process up through this juncture is something that is critically important as I reflect on leadership in nursing—something that is valuable and transportable. I learned that nurses work together and create networks with each other; they keep track of, support, and mentor each other. The network of nurses in academia was continually helping one another grow into the next phases of their careers. In short, they were working together to better their profession and engender the next generation of nursing leadership.

What is most striking about this is that the "helping" nature of the profession extended far beyond patient care; the effort to help others connected to students and colleagues and to me. Indeed, I was repeatedly struck by the lack of competitiveness among the nursing leaders I met. Each seemed genuinely interested in helping SVC find a leader, and they were not the least bit concerned about another program growing and succeeding. Acutely aware of the shortage of nurses and nursing faculty/leaders, they were willing to look beyond themselves and their institutions to assist their profession.

But what is equally impressive is that the nursing leaders I came to know not only heard what we were looking for but understood the role we wanted a new leader to play—the expanded role I described. And they embraced the concept of a leader moving across the disciplines; they appreciated, and I think respected, that need for nursing students to get more than "technical" nursing education. They understood that the liberal arts and sciences were of value. Perhaps this was more shocking to me than it should have been—perhaps I, along with others, misperceived how nurses think about their profession and the effort they have expended to change existing stereotypes of nurses and nursing education.

The candidates we were introduced to through the just-described network were, without exception, impressive and quite different each from the other. How beneficial that we were seeing candidates who had different styles, different strengths, different experiences. And, when we found the candidates we best liked, I turned to the network again, to think through the choices and the strengths and weaknesses of the candidates.

The candidate we chose spent a fair amount of time with me, exploring the role she would play. To be sure, she met with the faculty, and the provost, and the interim chair. But she heard me speak repeatedly about the SVC mission, about the role of nursing in a liberal arts and sciences college, about the ways in which I thought the nursing chair could and should participate in our larger community. She did not come from academia; she came from a hospital setting where she developed ongoing training programs and educational offerings for health care professionals. What she understood well were the skills needed to succeed in health care now and into the future—and she had an uncanny appreciation of the need for life long learning.

Our new chair took some time to transition from her former position to her new position, but we engaged her in all hiring decisions and end-of-academic-year events during this interim period. So when she took over her leadership role on August 1, 2011, she was not new to the SVC community or to her role. Indeed, she was ready to start—ready to lead.

MOVING FROM LESSONS LEARNED INTO ACTION

Some of the hardest lessons I learned through this process relate to the difficulty of crossing or bridging silos within an institution. In theory, at least, we know it is right to work with others in different disciplines. That is at the core of why we value the liberal arts and sciences. Indeed, the work we all do and that our graduates will do requires interaction among a host of disciplines, given our increasingly complex and specialized world. Most problems we try to solve in this world are not confined to one discipline, despite our best pigeonholing efforts. This is true in health care, in law, in the war on poverty, in education. But if we cannot get out of our own silo, then our capacity to work together is impaired.

We have an opportunity on campuses to remediate this issue; we can and should find more ways that faculties work together, coteaching courses, serving on committees, doing presentations on campus for students to see, sharing pedagogical strategies that work, coauthoring papers. We need to create opportunities to role model this behavior in formal and informal ways. This takes three essential ingredients: time, money, and will. It is vastly easier—albeit not better—to "bowl alone."

An example from the just-described search. We wanted all prospective chairs to make a presentation to our community. In this instance, I had hoped that, in addition to health care faculty and staff and health care students, there would be other nonhealth care members of our community in the audience. But, apart from some members of the Senior Leadership team, that did not occur, which only reinforced for me the need for our nursing faculty and the new chair to spread their wings beyond their departments to the institution as a whole. Indeed, the audience at the presentations was a living example of silos that existed on our campus and the need to eradicate them. Hiring a chair of any division should interest our entire community, not just the division doing the hiring. The fact that the presentation did not draw folks in droves reinforced for me the difficulty in silo busting. Even something as simple as how we label presentations sends a message. So if we identify an event as a "nursing presentation," it signals that only nursing students should attend. Ironically, the nursing chair candidate's presentation directly addressed how students across our institution could be enrolled together in courses that were cotaught with shared disciplinary expertise.

We owe it to our students—those in health care and those in other fields—to find greater avenues for them to engage together in and outside of the classroom. Divisional chairs and faculty can be role models for encouraging cross-pollination. Saying the right thing is not nearly enough. We need to do the right thing day in and day out on our campuses. Now, I appreciate that developing competencies even within one field is challenging enough, and there is no shortage of information that students need to learn, particularly in fields with licensing exams and a prescribed set of competencies to be mastered.

The next lesson I learned—about the shared commitment among nursing leaders to working together—led me to ponder ways we can get our nursing students to work together even more effectively, reducing the competition among them and enabling them to care not just for their patients but for each other. Indeed, that would be a useful skill set to develop among all of our students. As a recent *New York Times Magazine* article, "The Character Test" by Paul Tough, noted, success involves vastly more than knowledge acquisition; character matters.

This approach is consistent with an already deepening culture in which we seek ways to engender a greater sense of institutional responsibility that students play in each other's lives. Consider these examples: matching first-year students with an upper class mentor; designing a campus community dinner project in which students work not only with community families but also with each other to enhance their skills at having difficult conversations. We are working to make our athletic team captains more than "athletic" leaders but community-wide leaders. We are fostering more team projects in classes. We have developed and are developing norming campaigns that enable students to better align their choices with respect to alcohol, drugs, and sex to their own value systems.

The lessons learned also prompted me to reflect on how we actually think about and teach leadership within the academy. For me, this implicates the complex question of **where** we find leaders and **how** we develop leaders.

On the "where" question, we hired a nursing chair who did not come up through the traditional academic ranks. We hired someone with the skill sets needed to be a nursing leader within the academy despite the fact that she had not been in the academy for years. What this means, for nursing and other fields, is that we need to consider the qualities we want in a leader and recognize that they can be fostered in a wide range of settings of which the academy is but one. In other words, leadership skills are transportable from one setting to another.

I should have known this myself actually, as I came to a college presidency with what people politely termed a "nontraditional" resumé. If the theory is that you hire college presidents only from the ranks of vice presidents and provosts and sitting presidents, I would never have become a president. Becoming a president from a different route was, I was once told, like capturing lightning in a bottle.

But, that is just the point. It should not be so rare. We can find more ways to capture lightning, to find leaders in unconventional ways, and in nontraditional places. And we need to believe—and experience is a good teacher—that leadership skills are not discipline specific and can be carried across the borders. Otherwise, we will have both a shortage in and a stultification of leadership. We know that successful leadership—true leadership—involves risks and takes courage. The same can and should be said about hiring decisions: they involve risk and can require courage.

In terms of training leaders, we tend to take something of a narrow view here as well. I appreciate that there are courses on leadership; I taught one myself at SVC. We also create a cadre of student leaders based on their involvement in student organizations and clubs. But we can do even more by doing a better job of signaling that we are all leaders—students too. We all can make our communities (large and small) better. We all can voice ideas that will contribute to our collective well-being. Think about this point with respect to students. If we empower them to think about improving their education—what they are learning, how they are learning, and the environment in which they are learning—they can start to develop leadership skills. If we help students self-reflect and strategize about how to improve issues that are bothering them on and off campus, we are fostering leadership early and often. If we ask students to develop expectations (goals) and then help them measure their progress against those goals, we are developing leadership.

Another way of thinking about this is to recognize that leadership is not just the person at the proverbial top. Nor are future leaders always the ones marching up the traditional ladder. Creating opportunities for leadership and recognizing leadership—ah, that is the key!

CONCLUSION

In an interesting way, our search for a leader in nursing enabled me to think more effectively about leadership, and in the world of unintended consequences, made me a better leader. One could say that, by every measure then, our search for a new chair of nursing was a success.

Nursing Leadership Lessons:
An Association Executive's Perspective

Wylecia Wiggs Harris

Commentary
by Joyce J. Fitzpatrick

Harris shares her insights about nurse leaders based on more than 25 years of experience working with a number of professional organization leaders. She describes the leadership process as a facilitative one that engages others to achieve shared goals. Through this lens she describes the leadership actions of three nurse leaders and illustrates the different approaches that they have used and the various core components of successful leadership.

In presenting these examples of successful nurse leaders, Harris stresses that there are multiple approaches to leadership. She describes the pragmatic, ideological, and charismatic leaders through the exemplars that she presents. Within these differing approaches to leadership, she identifies the common success strategies. One of the most important characteristics of success is the leaders' orientation to others, ability to collaborate with others toward mutual goals, communication skills, and willingness to take risks.

Harris offers seven key lessons learned from her experiences and her analysis of nurse leaders. These include the advice to prepare oneself for leadership, through both educational and experiential learning; learn the political process and learn to use power in

> leadership roles; manage one's image, including all
> dimensions of the communication that is imparted
> by language, behavior, and attire; learn and practice
> socialized leadership, which necessitates involving
> others in the process; develop one's emotional intelli-
> gence through self-awareness and self-reflection; value
> authenticity and integrity and live these values; and
> be open to and embrace new ideas, opportunities, and
> challenges.
>
> One of the most important messages from Har-
> ris is that nurses and nursing organizations must
> focus on image management and rid themselves of
> the painful divisions that have plagued the profes-
> sion for so long. This advice must be heeded if nurses
> are going to influence health care in the future. We
> have heard this refrain many times; it is now time to
> act on it.

Key focus areas: collaborative partnerships, credibility, emotional
intelligence, image management, politically astute, values driven

The world of association management presents a unique opportunity to view nursing leaders in a variety of roles as they
transfer their skills and knowledge from the nursing profession to
their association leadership roles; and to view how they address
the challenges and opportunities presented by their volunteer leadership positions. Over the past 25 years, I have been fortunate to
work with a number of nursing leaders in my capacity as an association executive. My current position as a senior executive with a
professional nursing association affords me a wonderful vantage
point to interact with and observe nursing leaders from an array of
professional settings and to observe their leadership strengths and
opportunities for growth.

Although various conceptualizations of leadership abound,
my personal experiences suggest that leadership is a facilitative

process that engages others to achieve shared goals. My view of leadership is shaped by my interactions with a number of leaders from varied professional backgrounds, insights gained during my academic doctoral preparation, and my own experiences as a seasoned executive. During the past 25 years, on the basis of direct and indirect interactions, I have observed nursing leaders who have skillfully demonstrated the ability to engage others and leverage their personal strengths to move forward their leadership agendas. I have also witnessed otherwise very competent individuals struggle to either initiate the engagement process with others necessary to further their leadership agenda or to sustain the engagement process.

This chapter explores how three successful nursing leaders, using different leadership approaches, demonstrate traditional leadership attributes such as strategic vision; risk-taking and creativity; interpersonal and communication effectiveness; and inspiring and leading change. Furthermore, observations are offered on the level of emotional intelligence and behavioral integrity evidenced by the three leaders. Finally, the chapter discusses the opportunities and implications for both nursing leaders and those external to the profession to develop collaborative and transformative partnerships to advance quality health care.

LEADERSHIP PROFILES OF THREE SUCCESSFUL NURSING LEADERS

Taking an outsider's perspective and offering observations on how nursing leaders can develop successful strategies for more effective collaboration and partnership to advance and transform quality health care is simultaneously a tremendous honor and a daunting task. The observations offered must be grounded in reality, protect one's relationship with the individuals chosen to profile, and yet contribute meaningful insights that help increase the capacity of nursing leaders to effect change. The approach taken in this chapter is to use a leadership framework to (1) stress that there are multiple approaches to exemplary leadership; (2) identify common success strategies employed by three extremely competent, but different nursing leaders portrayed; and (3) offer a structure that may be useful to the readers of this book to personally evaluate to what degree they exhibit the characteristics of the three nursing leaders profiled.

To accomplish these objectives, I found it useful to frame my observations by reviewing three distinct pathways to leadership success: pragmatic, ideological, and charismatic leadership. These three pathways are well researched in the leadership literature, and the general observations shared are not unique. What is different than past conceptualizations of these three leadership pathways is the application of pragmatic, ideological, and charismatic leadership qualities to successful nursing leaders.

Nursing Leader A: Pragmatic Leader Profile

Pragmatic leaders demonstrate leadership excellence by effectively translating their nursing care assessment skills into the ability to approach organizational problem solving and decision making in a systematic, logical manner. A case in point is Nursing Leader A who effectively used her focus on fact-based decision making to achieve national prominence as a leader, which consequently earned her the right to sit at numerous decision-making tables to positively impact societal change.

Nursing Leader A entered nursing during a time of great societal unrest, and her competence as a nurse was questioned at every opportunity. Her prescription for overcoming resistance was to always be prepared. As such, knowledge and the ability to factually demonstrate a proposed course of action were instrumental in overcoming barriers to personal and organizational success. Leader A excels as a leader, unlike other individuals who may employ a pragmatic approach, because her use of a pragmatic leadership pathway results in a propensity for calculated risk taking and creative thinking. She has an uncanny ability to take complex issues and distill them down into manageable tasks to address issues. She values data and is most receptive to feedback that is couched in concrete evidence. This individual uses her analytical skills to both inform decision making and to engage others in the decision-making process. The ability to demonstrate a strong sense of self-awareness coupled with the capacity to motivate others is a strength for this individual. Although data driven, her search for concrete evidence makes her open to diverse ideas and people. Nursing Leader A is an effective communicator; however, equally important, she is politically savvy and possesses a high degree of behavioral integrity. Her current work environment requires that she interface with a diverse group of stakeholders with well-entrenched political agendas and egos. Her personal value system keeps her grounded in what is acceptable behavior. Her belief in documentation and evidence-based approaches has established her credibility and made it challenging for her detractors to hinder her effectiveness. Other pragmatic nursing leaders whom I have encountered possess many of the same characteristics attributed to Nursing Leader A, but have not achieved the same level of success.

What is the difference between Nursing Leader A and other nursing leaders who use a pragmatic leadership approach? Overlying how leaders make decisions and resolve problems is their orientation to others. They may consistently initiate actions to improve the collective welfare of the organization's various stakeholders. In contrast, they may consistently place their interests and welfare above the needs of others. Achieving personal dominance is the driving force behind the orientation of personalized leaders. One of the reasons for Nursing Leader A's success is that she places the interests of the organization above her own interests. As such, although she is less strategic than other leaders I have observed, her genuine interest in and concern for others enables her to sustain stakeholder engagement. This means she is able to form strong teams and leverage the strengths of others to achieve goals and objectives. As an individual who is open to input from others, she uses fact-based decision making to evaluate the best ideas presented by others. However, she is careful to acknowledge the contributions of others in the decision-making process. Integral to sustaining follower and stakeholder engagement is an awareness of how one's actions and feelings impact others and their job performance. A strong self-awareness supports the development of collaborative relationships. As a result, Nursing Leader A effectively builds and maintains collaborative relationships with both internal and external constituents. Finally, what distinguishes Nursing Leader A from other leaders in general is her behavioral integrity. There is congruence between her words and actions; and as such she is perceived as a credible leader. The lesson offered from the profile of Nursing Leader A is that being a cognitively strong leader is not sufficient to support collaborative relationships. Behavioral integrity, credibility, sustained stakeholder engagement, and high self-awareness of one's impact on others are important distinguishing factors that support collaborative dialogue and the establishment of the partnerships necessary to address complex issues.

A challenge faced by Nursing Leader A is her strong preference for concrete evidence. She is sometimes reticent to pursue
a course of action or recommend a solution without all the facts.
Informed decision making is critical; the key is making decisions
with enough data to ensure a reasonable probability of being right,
but not waiting until you have enough facts to ensure 100% accuracy. There are times when a decision must be rendered without
the benefit of a complete analysis in order to capitalize on potential
opportunities. Nursing Leader A may occasionally miss an opportunity because of her high data needs. Nursing leaders who tend
to rely on the concreteness and completeness of information must
recognize that this preference may sometimes impede the ability to
seize opportunities in a timely fashion.

Nursing Leader B: Charismatic Leader Profile

In contrast to the present-needs focus of pragmatic leaders, charismatic leaders are vision-based leaders who predicate their leadership agenda on attaining future goals. Charismatic leaders, perhaps
in part because of their natural charisma, are often portrayed as
successful or outstanding leaders. This general description of charismatic leaders holds true for Nursing Leader B. This individual
is personable and fully comprehends how to effectively communicate her personal vision in a compelling manner. When considering all the nursing leaders whom I have worked with or observed,
Nursing Leader B is one of the strongest leaders in terms of strategic
visioning and communication effectiveness. This individual is perceived by both internal and external organizational constituents as
a tenacious leader, engaging, and highly successful. She has effectively demonstrated her change agent abilities by shepherding her
organization through a period of intense turmoil, facilitating the
organization in achieving many of its organizational benchmarks,
and positioning the organization for future success. She uses both
her strong verbal skills and nonverbal behaviors to marshal individuals to pursue common organizational goals. She values and
orchestrates strategic partnerships and alliances that further her
personal, professional, and organizational objectives. Leader B is an
extremely inspiring communicator who effectively paints a picture
of the future to engage followers. She is a masterful storyteller and
understands the importance of influence and power. Storytelling

combined with humor and passion enables Nursing Leader B to build bridges of understanding across diverse stakeholder groups. She is a creative thinker, and risk taking is an integral component of her leadership approach. Further, she projects and protects her image of being a competent, politically astute leader.

Nursing Leader B is driven and passionate about her organization. Her drive and passion increase her personal strength as a leader; however, they also represent her Achilles heel. Although verbally open to diverse opinions and approaches, her passion and high drive sometimes convey a different message that suggests conformity to her approach or exclusion from the process. Her quest to ensure the long-term viability of her organization coupled with her strong character can initially hinder her ability to listen and entertain alternative approaches. Furthermore, the intense focus on achieving the vision that she has painted can lead her to consciously or subconsciously silence individuals who share a divergent perspective from her envisioned future. As a consequence, perhaps unknown to this leader, some individuals perceive the tactics used to achieve her objectives as too aggressive. This perception, whether or not accurate, can cast this leader as a personalized leader who is more focused on her personal agenda than the needs of the collective. Finally, Nursing Leader B's personal drive makes it difficult for this individual to publically acknowledge mistakes and to make amends.

Nursing Leader B is undoubtedly a strong strategic thinker, is creative, a risk-taker, and an effective communicator. The challenge faced by this leader is that she may not fully comprehend the extent of how her behaviors and actions affect others. Or, if she does on some level comprehend the effect, achieving the articulated vision may take a higher priority than the impact of her behaviors and actions on others. This may be an unfair assessment of an otherwise strong leader. However, the self-awareness of her actions affects the perception of her behavioral integrity as well as the effectiveness of her interpersonal skills. Both of these attributes are integral to building and sustaining viable partnerships.

Nursing Leader C: Ideological Leader Profile

There are several similarities between Nursing Leader B and Nursing Leader C, who, similar to Nursing Leader B, rose to leadership prominence in her organization during a period of turmoil and strife. Furthermore, like Nursing Leader B, Nursing Leader C is also a vision-based leader. The difference is that unlike Nursing Leader B's futuristic focus, Nursing Leader C's focus is rooted in past successes and traditions. Her diverse professional background, in terms of industry, clinical, and administrative positions held, has enabled her to hone her leadership skills, including the ability to effectively lead large-scale organizational change. This hardworking individual is a committed leader whose primary focus is to return her organization to a point of past glory and success. The primary strategy used by this individual to accomplish this goal is to allow her value system to inform her decision making, including the strategies employed for stakeholder engagement. As a values-driven leader, the core values that drive this individual are integrity, hard work, commitment, and loyalty. Furthermore, this individual is an articulate leader who recognizes the importance of honoring personal and organizational commitments.

As a leader often cast into leading organizational change in the midst of crisis, Nursing Leader C operates from a central command perspective versus a more facilitative, empowering leadership approach. She does not shy away from assuming visible leadership roles and is willing to leverage organizational resources to ensure that her organization is a prominent player at key decision-making tables. She demonstrates courage and risk-taking behavior and is willing to accept the consequences for decisions that may go awry. She is a decisive leader who treasures rituals and symbols.

The challenges faced by this individual center on her strong ideological bent and inability to hear and value individuals whose ideology may differ significantly from her own, the difficulty in shifting from a command and control leadership approach to a more facilitative leadership approach, and the political sophistication to know when the deck is stacked and it is time to walk away from a situation or an idea.

LESSONS LEARNED

As I reflect on these three nursing leaders and their successes, there are seven key lessons that can be derived from their experiences to enhance the ability of nursing leaders to engage in meaningful partnerships to advance transformative change.

Lesson 1: Be Prepared

Although Nursing Leaders A, B, and C use different primary leadership pathways, they share the common mindset of being prepared to lead. Preparedness can take several forms such as furthering one's formal education, mentoring, and coaching. It may also include volunteering for additional assignments in the workplace, professional association, or charitable activities that provide the opportunity to develop additional leadership skills and/or gain additional visibility and credibility. Equally important, preparation means building strategic networks within and external to the work environment to support one's leadership agenda and aspirations. Finally, preparation involves strategically thinking about their leadership abilities and their capacity to effect change within the current professional context and how best to position oneself to ensure the opportunity to participate in the right forums to advance change.

In the case of the three individuals profiled, all three individuals elected to advance their formal education, leveraged their involvement in work and professional association activities, and sought mentors as a strategy to build name recognition and credibility. These individuals value continuous learning and leverage this appetite for learning with their strong work ethic to develop a keen understanding of issues that confront their organizations and the collaborative partnerships in which they participate. Furthermore, they effectively use their knowledge and the power gained from being able to concisely articulate a particular stance to advance their leadership agendas and to position them to be considered for elevated opportunities. Recognizing that hard work and education would not be sufficient to ensure that their talents and capabilities were recognized, the three nursing leaders profiled began early in their careers to build personal and collegial networks to support their professional development and to help advance their leadership agendas. Strategic networks, especially informal networks, are important to career advancement. They help the leader obtain critical information not widely available to individuals participating in collaborative partnerships. Access to informal channels enables leaders to access information that can help guide them through or around political minefields and other barriers that might otherwise limit their leadership effectiveness.

Leaders who recognize the importance of preparedness as a key advancement strategy for their leadership agenda within organizations and collaborative partnerships (1) recognize their innate talents and potential as leaders, (2) address any developmental areas that could potentially impede their leadership credibility and effectiveness, (3) recognize that the right to be seated at the decision-making table must be earned by value-added contributions, and (4) identify strategies that enable them to successfully navigate the political landscape.

Lesson 2: Become Politically Astute and Effectively Use Power

Politics exist within all organizations and may be more prevalent as individuals advance the leadership ranks. The key is not to avoid politics, but to develop one's personal playbook for advancing an agenda that supports goal attainment within one's personal value system. Depending on the arena in which one leads or desires to lead, it may be important not only to be politically astute, but to bring political capital to the table that supports a collaborative partnership in achieving its partnership goals. Part of becoming politically astute is to understand the importance and role of power and influence.

Viewing power from an appropriate perspective can help nursing leaders more effectively build collaborative partnerships. Based on my observations, some nurses are uncomfortable with the concept of power when depicted in explicit or direct terms. However, this may be the primary approach to power used by others at the decision-making table. The inability to understand the time and place for using harsh versus soft power skills can disadvantage nurse leaders and limit their effectiveness. Likewise, the overuse of power in a manner that squelches collaboration can also hinder effectiveness.

Each of the three nursing leaders profiled understands the importance of being politically astute and effectively leveraging power and influence to make value-added contributions. In a dialogue with Nursing Leader A on how to develop political astuteness, she stressed the importance of understanding an organization's culture and seeking mentors who can help guide individuals through politically charged situations.

Lesson 3: Practice Image Management

It goes without saying that everyone does not have our best interests at heart and may not present our successes or failures in the
most favorable light. All leaders must work hard to build and sustain their leadership credibility and image. At times, nursing leaders may need to step out of their comfort zone to ensure that their
behaviors, language, personal leadership style, and attire support
and not distract from their educational credentials and leadership
competencies. It may be necessary to mirror or emulate the image
of what is considered a successful leader within a given environment to gain initial leadership credibility. This may be a difficult
lesson for some nursing leaders to accept. Unfortunately, depending on the leadership context, decisions related to credibility may
be based on how you look when you show up at the discussion
table and not only on what you can offer to advance the dialogue.

   My observation of the three individuals profiled is that they recognize the importance of image management and work hard to protect their leadership image. All three individuals guard the amount
of information they share about themselves personally to certain
audiences, remain focused on issues and not personality, emulate
the language and attire of the group with whom they are interacting,
consciously maximize photo opportunities with the right individuals, and leverage situations to demonstrate their individual strengths
and abilities to work within a collaborative partnership.

Lesson 4: Demonstrate Socialized Leadership

As a facilitative process, leadership requires that successful leaders
master how to maximize the productivity and contributions of others to achieve a common objective. Whether within the confines of
an organization or at the collaborative table for monumental issues
such as transforming health care, individuals who approach leadership from a socialized perspective will in the long term be better
able to sustain the engagement process necessary to find common
ground to address issues. Although some may disagree with this
perspective, I have witnessed competent leaders who are creative, effective communicators, resourceful, risk takers, and strategic thinkers experience derailment in their careers because of the
inability to sustain the engagement process. Somewhere along their
leadership trajectory, they became more focused on the needs of

self versus the needs of the collective, and the resulting outcome was a loss of leadership credibility. Focusing on the good of the collective does not imply that leaders should be self-sacrificing and never make decisions that advance their own career opportunities. Rather, socialized leaders acknowledge that their advancement is predicated on service to others and in partnership of seeking common ground. Furthermore, they recognize that once credibility and behavioral integrity are damaged, it is difficult to rebuild trust. Examples of leaders within a variety of areas such as sports, politics, entertainment, business, and even nursing underscore that personalized leadership in the long run can be extremely detrimental to the individual leader and organizational unit led by the individual.

To varying degrees, the various constituents of the three nursing leaders profiled view them as socialized leaders. In the case of Nursing Leaders B and C, unconscious behaviors contributed to perceptions by some of their constituents that their leadership approach tilted toward personalized leadership. And, although this perception must be balanced with the political climate in which these individuals lead their organizations, it is important to note that maintaining a socialized leadership orientation takes hard work and consistency.

Lesson 5: Develop High Emotional Intelligence

Historically, strong interpersonal and social skills represent a characteristic of successful leaders. The three nursing leaders profiled in this chapter each possess strong interpersonal skills and a comfort interacting with individuals at various organizational and social levels. However, in today's complex and increasingly culturally diverse environments, leaders must possess not only strong interpersonal/social skills but a high degree of overall emotional intelligence. Self-awareness, self-regulation, motivation, empathy, and social skills are key components of emotional intelligence that enable leaders to gauge how their actions are impacting others and modulate their behaviors as necessary. Why is this important to nursing leaders? Being able to take their critical thinking and assessment skills and apply them in diverse arenas represents a key advantage for nursing leaders. However, to fully capitalize on this advantage, nursing leaders must modify their leadership approach and behaviors based on their assessment of the given leadership situation. They must do this in a manner that enables them to be true to their core values while recognizing that different situations may require different approaches. It is insufficient to assess only the situation or problem; they must also be able to assess how their own behavior may contribute to or hinder collaborative efforts and adjust their behaviors accordingly. Equally important, nursing leaders must understand how to leverage their strengths and values effectively to ensure the inclusion of perspectives important to their constituents when participating in collaborative activities. For example, Nursing Leader A combines her strong interpersonal skills with her evidence-based approach to ensure that she (1) understands the needs of all the players involved in a collaborative endeavor and (2) presents the case for support of her ideas in a manner that can be heard and generally accepted by others. Likewise, Nursing Leader B recognizes that her directness can sometimes be interpreted as abrasiveness and leverages her humor and storytelling ability to build linkages with others and to find areas of common agreement. Nursing Leader C uses her values to inform how she interacts with others and to ensure that her integrity and work ethic are evident in her dealings with collaborative partners. However, as previously noted in the case of Nursing Leaders B and C, even successful leaders with high emotional intelligence can be slow to recognize when their behavior and actions are out of step within a given leadership context.

Lesson 6: Value and Exhibit Integrity and Authenticity

Increased disillusionment and distrust is an outcome of high-profile organizational scandals, broken political promises, a widening gap between the haves and have-not's, and continued division on a host of social and political issues. It is against this colorful backdrop that nursing leaders and others interested in transforming health care must find common ground and moral courage to effect positive, sustainable change. Leaders who are competent, confident in their abilities, and principle-centered can operate from a vantage point that enables them to help others rise above the fray and remain focused on the common goals of the collaborative effort. Yet, maintaining integrity and authenticity in the midst of heated discussions and underhanded politics is sometimes challenging.

By their own admissions, Nursing Leaders A, B, and C are all faith-centered individuals. Although manifested in different ways, their faith is an integral component of their personal identity and shapes their values perspective and proposition. Each of these leaders have faced challenges to their values and from their vantage point have remained true to what they value. Consequently, while others may not always agree with their decisions, they do generally respect what these individuals have accomplished as leaders. However, these leaders recognize that their wonderful accomplishments and accolades may be quickly forgotten if lapses in integrity and authenticity occur and are detected by others.

Lesson 7: Be Open to New Ideas and Opportunities

Reflecting on the lives and experiences of the three nursing leaders profiled in this chapter, each was positioned to participate in national leadership dialogues because they were open to new ideas and new opportunities. It is easy to become stagnant and rest on the laurels of past successes; however, it is the willingness to shift gears as necessary and pursue new horizons that enables individuals to take advantage of unprecedented opportunities to influence and shape widespread organizational and/or societal change.

IMPLICATIONS FOR LEADERS INTERNAL
TO THE NURSING PROFESSION

Nursing is uniquely positioned not only to participate in transformative and collaborative partnerships to advance quality health care, but to provide the leadership necessary to accomplish this daunting task. The sheer number of nurses within the country makes the nursing profession a formidable force for change. The challenge faced by nursing is the internal divisions that limit the ability to galvanize the entire nursing community to present a united front and capitalize on its collective power. This fracturing within the nursing community may impede the ability of nursing leaders to build transformative and collaborative partnerships if multiple nursing leaders sit at the discussion table each with a different agenda and perspective on how to represent nursing in the process. The nursing community and its leaders must learn to privately disagree on matters and still be able to develop a cohesive external approach that enables a variety of nursing leadership representatives to engage in transformative dialogues with a commonality of purpose.

The seven lessons offered for individual nursing leaders are also germane to the nursing community as the profession rightfully seeks to participate in dialogues to advance quality health care. For example, the nursing community must be prepared with a common agenda or vision for the role of nursing to engage in collaborative conversations, and it must ensure the best prepared, most knowledgeable, and politically astute individuals sit at the table to represent the interests of the nursing profession and the patients they serve. The vetting process of those nursing leaders recommended to serve on collaborative partnerships should be intentional, based on identifying the most qualified nursing representatives for the particular leadership opportunity, and reach beyond established nursing networks to include nursing leaders external to mainstream nursing organizations. These nursing representatives may emerge from different practice settings, participate as members of different professional nursing associations, have different political affiliations, and may have different perspectives on how to recruit and retain a healthy nursing workforce; however, there needs to be a common agenda that cuts across these differences and enables these representatives to present a unified nursing front on advancing quality health care. Preparation further includes developing a national cadre of emerging nursing leaders and nurse-friendly advocates who are mentored, coached, and positioned to assume prominent positions of leadership in key local, state, regional, and national partnerships.

Finally, nursing as a profession needs to practice image management. Early in my career, I was oblivious to the internal strife that exists within the nursing profession. I hold nurses and the nursing profession in the highest regard. However, I am now aware of some of the painful divisions that separate the nursing community and fear that these painful divisions will become more apparent to those external to the nursing community and begin to erode the positive image of nursing among the general public. Nursing should, at all costs, protect its professional image and leverage its positive image to make it difficult for conveners to consider a local, state, or national dialogue on health care that does not include the multifaceted voice of nursing.

IMPLICATIONS FOR LEADERS EXTERNAL TO THE NURSING PROFESSION

Any dialogue related to advancing quality health care will be incomplete and off base without the active participation of nursing leaders and cannot be considered a collaborative process. A truly collaborative dialogue must be interdisciplinary in nature and include either directly or indirectly the voice of the consumer. Nursing represents a critical linchpin in the health care delivery system and as such can offer insights regarding the need for systemic changes that support quality health care. Recognizing the importance of the nurses' voice in the dialogue, external leaders committed to the collaborative process and a positive outcome should ensure that nurses are invited to participate in local, state, regional, and national partnerships. However, beyond providing the opportunity for participation, external leaders can help mentor and coach nursing leaders on how to most effectively position themselves and the profession in the dialogue so that their important perspective can be heard. Furthermore, external leaders should avoid the practice of tokenism and ensure that adequate numbers of nursing leaders are slotted in dialogue forums consistent with the size of the nursing constituency.

CONCLUDING THOUGHTS

An external perspective on nursing leadership must be couched in the reality that observers cannot fully comprehend the complexity and challenges of the nursing profession and the individuals who serve as its leaders. The lessons offered in this chapter, based on the three nursing leaders profiled, are intended to support the overall dialogue on increasing the individual and community capacity of nurses to serve as collaborative partners to transform and advance quality health care. It takes moral courage for leaders to look in the mirror and reflect on the things they do well and the things they need to improve to increase their overall effectiveness. As a consumer of health care services and as an individual who firmly believes in the importance of nurses participating in an interdisciplinary approach to shape care delivery systems, I encourage current and aspiring nursing leaders to thoughtfully reflect on the outsider perspectives offered on nursing leadership in this book. Take from this book what is relevant to help you grow and become a transformational leader well positioned to participate in and lead collaborative dialogues on advancing quality health care.

11

Philanthropy and Nursing Leadership

Kate Judge

Commentary
by Joyce J. Fitzpatrick

Judge makes a compelling case for nursing leader-ship through philanthropy. She aptly describes the role of the leader as one who can communicate a compelling reason to invest in the power of nursing as a key to quality in health care. Accordingly, the nurse leader in this arena must develop a set of skills that at one level goes beyond the traditional nursing skill set, but at the same time is grounded in key nursing skills of communication; relationship building; and interest in the values, hopes, and ideals of others, the donors.

The essential characteristics of the nurse leader in philanthropy that Judge delineates are the ability to focus on a greater good; a commitment to building solutions, including both an immediate impatience and long-term perspective of the solution; clarity and constancy of message; the ability to compel and attract potential donors; the ability to embrace a larger world; willingness to be known by others; and skill at devel-oping relationships.

Judge presents a positive message, one that is instructive for all nurse leaders who can build and enhance their nursing foundational skills to advance the larger professional and societal goals of improv-ing the lives of others. Nurses and nurse leaders are everywhere, representing 1% of the U.S. population.

> *Thus, according to Judge, in developing their leader-*
> *ship skills in philanthropy, nurse leaders can poten-*
> *tially capture 1% of the $298 billion given annually*
> *to nonprofit organizations in the United States. This*
> *is an important agenda and goal for the greater good*
> *of nursing and health care.*

Key focus areas: moral purpose, consistent and compelling communication, sustained attraction, embrace a larger world, relationship building

My first glimpse of nursing leadership in action came the day I arrived at the University of Pennsylvania School of Nursing for an in-person interview to lead Penn Nursing's development and alumni relations program. It was clear from meeting both faculty and staff that they saw their work at Penn within the larger context of advancing health. For example, the Penn Nursing admissions staff wanted to attract, admit, and yield the best and brightest students. All admissions departments are tasked similarly. Their success would bring honor to Penn Nursing with a distinguished entering class with high GPAs. But their commitment went beyond what would be a great ranking statistic for Penn. They were passionate and unendingly creative about how to recruit students who would be the women and men who could change health care overall. That is leadership.

This commitment to a good beyond one's own interest is a personal value that brought me to philanthropy as a career. I have spent the past 25 years leading fund-raising and communication programs for both large and small nonprofit organizations. I have worked with faculty and staff to secure gifts from individuals, corporations, and foundations for scholarships, educational programs, technology, basic research, health care delivery, endowed scholarships, and disaster relief.

Most of my professional fund-raising has been in academia, first as a director of development at the University of Wisconsin and then as an assistant dean at the University of Pennsylvania. Today,

I am an executive director of the American Nurses Foundation, a nurse-focused charity, which I joined because of the inspirational nurse leaders I met at Penn.

During my 8 years at Penn Nursing, I collaborated with a number of faculty members who were gifted in attracting philanthropy. Professor Ellen Baer turned an impromptu meeting with a friend of a friend at a New York restaurant into one of the largest nursing scholarship programs in the United States. Dean Norma Lang's passion for nursing, down-to-earth approach, and ability to both predict and translate health care's evolution enabled her to make deep connections with donors and secure funding for endowed professorships and innovative nurse-managed practices. Dean Emeritus Claire Fagin, also the first woman president of an Ivy League institution, demonstrated what I consider one of the greatest acts of leadership in philanthropy—an example that inspires me still. While she was dean at Penn's School of Nursing, she helped secure eight endowed chairs for Penn and seven *other* schools of nursing. She was most clearly focused upon the greater good.

When a dean draws a picture for prospective donors about the importance and power of a donor's gift, she (or he) should be expansive—even global—in describing impact, but the financial focus must always be local: "Give to my institution to make a lasting difference." In the ever more competitive world of academic fund-raising, a dean is competing with other institutions or charities for each and every dollar raised. This milieu makes Claire's work with Philadelphia-based Independence Foundation to create eight endowed chairs most remarkable.

When I asked her why she had helped raise so many endowed chairs for other institutions—which I believe had never been done before or since by a dean of an institution—she said, "I knew they weren't going to endow more than one chair at Penn. But I understood from listening to them that they wanted to change the direction of their funding and do something substantial in education. What could be more important than nursing?"

In focusing on a greater good, Claire's leadership guided much needed financial capital to academic nursing. Perhaps even more important, she provided leadership capital to the seven other deans of schools of nursing *and*, at the same time, raised the stature and visibility of nursing as an academic philanthropic target nationally.

Nursing and philanthropy are relatively new partners. As I write this, private philanthropy in the United States contributes

$298 billion **annually** to nonprofits. Those dollars enable people to eat, have shelter, learn, teach, farm, raise children, be safe, create, recover, and be cured. Although nursing receives less than one thousandth of those contributions, today its share is increasing dramatically.

In the past 20 years, academic nursing has attracted unprecedented amounts of private support. Through the leadership of presidents, deans, faculty, and professional fund-raising staff, philanthropic support has grown from endowing scholarships for $10,000, to endowing professorships for $3,000,000, to endowing entire programs and new schools.

In addition to long-standing nursing funders, such as the Robert Wood Johnson Foundation, John A. Hartford Foundation, and the Helene Fuld Health Trust, there are new donors like Betty and George Gordon Moore, whose $100 million gift launched the School of Nursing at University of California–Davis; Donald and Barbara Jonas, who made a $100 million investment in the Jonas Center for Nursing Excellence to support nursing doctoral study; the Rita and Alex Hillman Foundation, whose commitment of over $39 million supports entry nursing education and bachelor of science in nursing (BSN) to PhD programs; Frank and Carol Morsani, who have given $37 million to the University of South Florida's School of Nursing; and J. Michael and Christine Pearson, whose $15 million gift to name the Duke School of Nursing's building.

When people write about leadership in philanthropy, they typically write about donors. Yet there are leaders on both sides of the philanthropic coin—those who lead through giving and those who lead by getting others to give. My focus on leadership in nursing is on the other side of the philanthropy equation—the getter versus the giver. Nurses' ability to inspire philanthropy—major philanthropy—is all about leadership.

Leadership in philanthropy combines a deep personal moral purpose and the perfect balance between impatience for immediate impact and a desire to achieve long-term outcomes. It requires a commitment to building solutions—whether they be made of bricks and mortar, like a hospital or library, or implementing strategies to eradicate a disease—that achieve a societal good extending beyond the life of the builder, donor, and planner. Leadership requires focus on results today *and* tomorrow.

The ability to lead in fund-raising must include **attraction**. Leaders draw others into their vision. I am not speaking about simple charisma. It is about sustained attraction that sets one above the noise of competing interests, organizations, and priorities. A leader must be able to strategically draw the right people—the right team—together to move something important forward. Whether it is recruiting the right student applicants, or collaborating with other professionals, or funders, people have to believe in a leader and trust in her (or his) ability and capacity to move the vision forward.

A leader must have a **clarity and constancy of message**. Claire Fagin communicated a consistent message about giving: It is logical, it is the right thing to do, it will be gratifying and rewarding to you as the donor, and people will truly benefit from your generosity. If nurses are to be successful fund-raisers, they must communicate effectively, regularly, and broadly about why nursing is the best, and in many ways most, desirable solution to health care issues.

A leader must be **compelling**. This requires combining the ability to engage others, to frame one's work and activities in a positive way, and to connect with those who are critical to accomplishing one's goals. The old adage that body language is 90% of a successful presentation is true about securing philanthropy; it is not the words in the proposal or case statement that raise money; it is the presentation that illuminates the meaning behind the words.

In addition to clear, consistent, and compelling communication about nursing, a nurse leader must be able to communicate about what others—donors, business leaders, social influencers—value and know. A leader must be willing to venture into social circles of wealth that can sometimes be intimidating, and be able to find common ground for a real conversation. To be a nurse leader in philanthropy, one must expose oneself to other values, interests, and priorities. Claire would readily tell you that she learned to work a room and learned about what others were interested in—art, business, literature. Leaders **embrace a larger world.**

A leader in philanthropy will set priorities and devote adequate time to accomplishing them. Success in philanthropy cannot be "jobbed out"—delegated solely to staff and volunteers. It demands persistence and investment of personal and organizational time. Leaders convey by the amount of time they themselves devote to philanthropy how they value donors' time and resources.

A leader's clarity in communication also relates to the **ability to be known by others**. Claire Fagin had an essential understanding of herself and communicated clearly who she was and what she wanted to accomplish. Leaders do not distract the people around them by causing them to wonder: "What does the leader mean or want? Who are they? What do they think?"

Claire was also refreshingly honest. This set her apart. It conveyed a comfortable **confidence**—essential for a leader to communicate persuasively. Donors invest their dollars when they feel that their monies are in good hands. Confidence is essential to trust, and trust is essential to philanthropy.

A leader practices and learns from mistakes. I have worked with several executives who were not willing to practice asking for money. They assumed that if they were strong communicators they could simply "talk" a solicitation. Rarely did they do it well.

Being willing to practice, like admitting mistakes, involves taking a risk. Leaders are risk-takers. They are bold in their vision and strategies and use their power of attraction to enlist others in their boldness. They provoke and cultivate a "yes we can" momentum. Claire's audacity to suggest endowing eight chairs in nursing at one time was a risk that paid off.

Finally, I believe leaders win the devotion of those around them by prioritizing and nurturing relationships. Attraction is not enough. A leader must draw people in and then **build relationships**. Claire made lasting relationships with donors, colleagues, and staff that won their loyalty and trust.

If nursing is to continue to expand its philanthropic appeal and impact, there must be more nurse leaders like Claire Fagin. It is interesting to note that although Claire is known as an innovator, a glass-ceiling breaker, an attractive role model, a strategic influencer—descriptions related to leadership skills and behaviors—little attention within nursing has been paid to her success in generating philanthropic support for nursing. **Her success in philanthropy serves as a** blueprint for describing nursing leadership in philanthropy for the future.

Nursing can assume a larger role in tomorrow's health care delivery if it commands a larger portion of U.S. and global philanthropy. Donors must experience more confidence from and about nurses and what nursing brings to the table. Nurses must make "what nurses do" compelling. They must engage in the power of attraction. Philanthropic giving is not an obligation due to nursing or nurses. It is not a "have-to"; it is a "want-to." People move toward what is bright, dynamic, strong, and colorful—toward what is transformative.

Finally, to be leaders in philanthropy, nurses need to educate themselves about the larger world and the values and issues that resonate with donors. Donors are more educated, inquisitive, and strategic in their philanthropic decision making than ever before.

Nurses in leadership roles in academia have demonstrated their understanding of the important role fund-raising plays in their institutions and careers. They have spent increasing amounts of time building relationships with donors—individuals, foundations, and corporations, who can invest in nursing education, research, and practice. It has paid off in hundreds of millions of dollars.

Leadership in nursing philanthropy needs to move beyond academia. The next phase is for nurses in other leadership roles and settings to accept the challenge of learning about, prioritizing, and attracting philanthropy. Individuals give the vast majority of the $298 billion in annual charity. Nurses touch the majority of those people every year in one way or another. Registered nurses constitute 1 out of every 100 people in the United States—1%. If nursing could achieve the same ratio in philanthropy there would be $2.98 billion *every* year to transform the world's health through the power of nursing. Claire Fagin would call that leadership.

12

Nursing Leadership: A View From Congress

Steven C. LaTourette

Commentary
by Joyce J. Fitzpatrick

*A*s a former member of the U.S. Congress and co-chair of the Nursing Caucus in the U.S. House of Representatives, LaTourette addresses the role nurses can and should provide in shaping national policy. The fact that nurses are consistently ranked among the trusted professionals in the eyes of the public puts them in a good negotiating position with legislatures, particularly when it comes to issues of health care.

Yet how many nurses even know that nurses have consistently been ranked as the most trusted professionals in the public's view? It is important for nurse leaders to make certain that this fact is understood by all nurses, as it would be both empowering and confidence building in the day-to-day work of the nurse, but also might encourage nurses everywhere to assume more active leadership roles.

LaTourette advises us that it is the relationship that elected representatives have with their constituents that drives the policy decision, not money or partisanship, particularly on issues such as nursing education. Nurses need to consistently develop relationships with their elected representatives. Yet we know from both the formal and informal analyses of nurses' involvement in political activity that only a small percentage are informed and involved. This must change for nurses to be at the center of health *care change. The nursing profession must engage a more significant percentage of its constituents to be influential. With more than 3 million nurses in the United States, the potential influence is great. As LaTourette recommends, to be leaders in the policy development process, nurses must understand the process. They must know the audience and build a trusting relationship with the policy maker and key members of his or her staff. Furthermore, it is important to each legislator that the message be delivered by a nurse in his or her voting body, not just by a national organization, no matter how representative the organization might be. LaTourette also advises that the nursing profession, and the many organizations that represent nursing, should be united in their messages to the legislators. And as he concludes, anything worth doing is worth doing right. Nurses need to get the political and policy process right.*

Key focus areas: speak with a single voice, relationships, learn the process, know your audience

For the last several sessions of the Congress, I have had the pleasure of being the Republican co-chair of the Nursing Caucus in the House of Representatives. Throughout that entire time I have had the honor of working with the Democratic co-chair, Lois Capps of California. Lois is a nurse by training, and I find myself always behind the learning curve because of her knowledge, education, and training, but I do the best I can to catch up. The trick to catching up is receiving good, reliable information from the stakeholders, the nurses, which dovetails nicely into writing about nursing leadership from the legislator's perspective.

I need to explain initially why I came to be involved in nursing issues. I dated for many years a woman who would later become very prominent in the nursing world. Our relationship began on our eighth-grade field trip to Washington, DC and continued through high school in Cleveland. After graduation, she attended the University of Michigan and I attended Case Western Reserve University on a scholarship. As is the case with most, but certainly not all, high-school romances, my head was filled more with ideals than common sense. I purchased a 1964 MGB with a body held together with more bondo than metal and would travel to Ann Arbor from Cleveland most weekends. Finding this arrangement less than satisfying, I decided to surrender my scholarship, transfer to Michigan, and pay out-of-state tuition. Needless to say, my parents were less than impressed with my choice and indicated that their participation in my college finances was over. So I amassed tens of thousands of dollars in student loans. I did not care, I was in love. Happy as a clam at high tide, I sailed through my undergraduate years. However, on the day we graduated, the girl dumped me. Not that I remember it very well, but on May 1, 1976, I had my degree but no girl, no car, and no money.

Fast forward 18 years, and my party approached me about running for Congress. I was opposing a Democratic incumbent, and you may remember one of the hot issues in the election in 1994 was health-care reform championed by President Clinton and the First Lady, Hillary Clinton. My opponent had a health care advisor to whom he turned for counsel, and his information was always first-rate. His advisor? That's right, the girl who dumped me.

So, I guess it is a fair question as to why I would even like nurses, let alone champion their causes on Capitol Hill. The answer is that, despite this woman's poor judgment in matters of the heart, the importance of the nurse in the care, treatment, and recovery of so many of my friends and neighbors made it a no-brainer.

That brings me to Congress and the leadership role that nurses can and should provide in shaping national policy.

There are a number of misconceptions about how policy is formed and influenced in Washington. Those misconceptions are driven by a skeptical public, a cynical media, a divisive political process and, yes, a few rotten apples who get elected. When they do public opinion surveys, it is always a contest to see which profession is least respected. We celebrate on Capitol Hill when members of Congress edge past attorneys and always know that the basement position will be occupied by used-car salesmen. Doctors and nurses, in contrast, always score near the top of the most trusted professions and that simple fact should put nurses in a strong position to advance their ideas. As an aside, only dentists fail to consistently score near the top, and, well, we all know why that is.

The first misconception is that money drives Washington. Although not completely without some truth, that belief is a gross oversimplification. Certainly, each of the nation's two major political parties has its large donor groups. For Republicans, it tends to be business interests and the Chamber of Commerce; for Democrats, labor and attorneys. However, the suggestion that campaign contributions are the sole driving force behind policy decisions is insulting to both the Congress and our constituency. The notion that a member of Congress would advance a position he or she does not believe is right to secure a $5,000 PAC (political action committee) check is nuts. I would posit that it is relationships that make the difference in Congress, and while attending a fundraiser may get you a few minutes of face time, it would not get your position adopted. Quite frankly, it is one of the reasons that the medical profession stinks at lobbying.

I can vividly remember when doctors were all focused on medical malpractice reform. Apparently, they had seen some protests on TV and decided they would organize marches on member's district offices to make their case. My office in Painesville, Ohio, is around the block from Lake East Hospital, and at the appointed time, 50 or so lab-coated physicians filed down the street from the hospital toward my office. Someone had also obviously observed that chants were appropriate as you storm the castle in outrage. Sadly, they forgot to tell the docs. So, while a number of these skilled surgeons, family care doctors, and anesthesiologists chatted on their cell phones, the "protest leader" with a bullhorn yelled out—"What do we want?" Which was greeted by a long silence and then a few brave voices responded—"tort reform." The leader queried—"When do we want it?" and those few brave souls guessed aloud—"Now?" Needless to say, medical malpractice reform has not happened. Similarly, in 2010 when the Affordable Care Act was being developed, it was big news that the AMA (American Medical Association) endorsed the health care bill. Again, remembering that the medical profession is held in high esteem by the public, this was a big deal. The sweetener for their support was a promise that the bill would finally fix the sustainable growth rate (SGR) and avoid a 21% cut in Medicare reimbursement slated for the beginning of 2011. Well, a funny thing happened on the way to bill passage. The promoters of the bill received a score from the Congressional

Budget Office that the so-called "doc fix" would cost in excess of $300 billion over the next decade. Already chagrined by the size of the bill, 2,000 pages, and a cost of $1 trillion, guess what happened to the doctors' sweetener? That's right, it was dropped.

This might be a good time to talk about partisanship and the need to reach consensus if you want your issue to prevail. As I mentioned earlier, Washington is a partisan place and some groups feel more comfortable having one party or the other serve as their champion. On issues that do not need to be partisan, like nursing education, it is a huge mistake to hitch your wagon to one party and ignore the other. One of the nice things about the Nursing Caucus is that partisanship stops at the water's edge when Lois and I discuss nursing. In the House of Representatives that can be especially important. I was elected in 1994 and became part of the first Republican majority in the House since 1954. The House is very much a "winner take all" place. The majority party controls what bills are considered, what amendments can be considered, and pretty much everything else. Being in the minority in the House is often referred to as the Mushroom Caucus, kept in the dark and fed manure. Well, we did such a great job that the voters tossed us out in the 2006 elections and the Democrats once again became the majority. As you know, the public's shelf life of patience appears to be shortening and the Republicans were the majority party after the elections of 2010 and 2012. President Obama was re-elected in 2012, and who knows what the public will be thinking and who will be in charge in 2015? The point is those groups that put it all on Republican Red in 1995 and made their issue a partisan pitch probably didn't do so well under the Pelosi speakership. Likewise, those who bet the house on the Pelosi speakership lasting more than 4 years have also needed to adjust their strategy. If your issue does not need to be a partisan one, do not let it become one. If you treat members from both parties evenly and fairly, you will do better in moving your cause.

Which brings me back to relationships and effective legislative leadership by nurses and other medical professionals. My first foray into nursing legislation came as a result of a single letter from a nurse at the Veterans Administration (VA) Hospital in Cleveland. Congress had earlier adopted locality pay schedules for VA nurses that were designed to increase nursing salaries: a noble goal since a large number of VA nurses were, at the time, on average 55 years of age and women. However, by the law of unintended consequences, because the law gave regional VA directors flexibility in setting nurses' pay, in times of tight budgets where they had no discretion in spending on other things, the law was used to retard or completely ignore any salary increases for the nursing staff. Although all other VA employees were seeing annual increases of 3% to 4%, nurses received less, and in some cases, no increases for years. By the time the nurse's letter hit my desk, some VA nurses had been without an increase for 5 years. As a result of that one letter, legislation was drafted that corrected the problem. It was bipartisan and sailed through to the President's desk for signature.

That same story has been repeated time and again on issues dealing with mandatory overtime, nursing faculty and education, anesthesia authorities, and a host of other issues. So why did the VA nurse succeed where the doctors' march failed?—relationships and a connection to the part of the country I represent. So the first failing that nurses, and others, make in attempting to shape policy is they do not take the time to learn the process and how best to advance their cause. I would not presume to come to a hospital and tell the medical professionals how to treat their patients for a number of reasons, one of them being that I have never studied the procedures. The same is true of the strange world of Congress. Most of us were schooled in a rudimentary course in how a bill becomes a law, but how many of you really know?

First, you need to know your audience. Why should I care about what it is you want to accomplish? The first step is the relationship and the next the message. If you do not trust the messenger, how can you trust the message? I am not talking about sending in my best friend to talk to me about nursing education, and certainly not the girl who dumped me. Although I have met many lovely nurses from all across the country, I am very interested in talking to a nurse from the Cleveland Clinic, Lake Hospital Systems, Summa, or University Hospitals. Why? Because those nurses are from where I am from and the people they care for are the people whom I represent. Next is trust. I see hundreds of people a week and all of them give me their views, ideas, and suggestions. The person or group that gives me good information will be turned to as a resource; the ones who come in to spin are not invited back. Last, you need to know what you are asking for and how it can be accomplished if I agree that it is a good idea.

Every year over 10,000 "great" ideas are drafted into bills submitted in the Congress. Only about 300 of those will ever become law. Learning the difference between "must pass" legislation and the bill that will be introduced to get you off my back is critical. The most fundamental "must pass" legislation are the Appropriation bills, and we do not always get those done. By contrast, bills authorizing some new program do not often fare so well. For instance, the State Department of the United States has never been authorized, so the chances of getting a nurse-specific piece of legislation authorized is challenging at best. Even if it gets through both houses of Congress and is signed by the President, if the appropriators do not put money behind it, there is no program. The art of effective leadership at the federal level is a little bit like going to a foreign country. Things go a lot more smoothly when you know the customs, practices, and language of the place you are visiting.

I do not mean any of the above to be criticism of the national nursing organizations that lobby the Hill. The ANA (American Nursing Association) and others do a nice job in knowing how the place works and are honest brokers that we turn to as resources on nursing issues. What they lack, however, is the connection to "home" that can only be supplied by putting, in my case, a Cleveland, Ohio, face on the issue. My suggestion is that before a nursing leader from "home" marches on the Hill, she or he takes some time to learn from the ANA or others how what she or he wants can get done.

Another one of Washington's secrets is that the staff really runs the place. Each member of Congress does his or her best to be knowledgeable on a host of issues. During the course of a week, the average member will cast 50 votes, see 50 appointments, attend 3 committee or subcommittee hearings and have a host of other meetings, calls, and briefings. Any member who claims he or she knows everything about every issue is either superhuman or fibbing. Developing a solid relationship with the member's staff is also a really good idea. The DC staff is divided by issue areas, and someone in each office will have your issue. Telling the person who answers the phone what it is you want done probably does not work really well. Discovering and forming a relationship with the appropriate staffer can lead to not only your issue making it into the member's briefing book but also saves you a trip to DC. From the comfort of your home you can call or e-mail the staffer and accomplish your purpose. While I am on the subject of staff, I would return to the old adage that you catch more flies with honey than vinegar. Nothing drives me crazier than some advocate calling and reading the riot act to one of my legislative assistants and demanding to talk to me. Almost always, when I get the rude individual on the phone, butter would not melt in this person's mouth. The caller is often courteous and demure. Why do some people think it is okay to treat a young person, probably in his or her first real job, rudely, when he or she is not the person making the decision, and then treat me like royalty?

Although every office runs a little differently, getting to know the staffer who handles your issue and treating him or her like a human being would not hurt. In my office, at the moment, nursing issues are handled by a lovely woman named Sarah. Sarah is from Ohio, is a graduate of Miami University, and attends law school at night. Her dad is a judge back home, and she hopes to follow in his footsteps when she is done with school. It would take you about 10 minutes of talking with Sarah to find those things out, and the next time you call you might have more to talk about. Sarah is responsible for contributing to my daily briefing book with the other legislative staff and if you have taken the time to get to know her, your issue will probably wind up as something for me to consider. If you treat Sarah like it is beneath you to talk to her, your issue may still wind up in my briefing book but a snowball probably has a greater chance of survival in Hades. The staff can also be a resource for how the Congress works and assist you in going from great idea to great law.

The second failure to punch through a nursing message is one that is not unique to nurses. Remembering that only 300 bills out of 10,000 will succeed, it is vital, where possible, to speak with a single voice. Let me stop picking on nurses for a minute to make the point. Kent State University is a wonderful college in Ohio with a good nursing program and several satellite campuses, two of which are in my district. Over the course of the year, I will be visited by Kent's president and, separately, by the deans of the satellites, the librarian, and the dean of the nursing school. In some years, I will receive 10 to 12 different things that the Kent State family wants from Congress. Most all are worthy, but Kent State is but one of a number of worthy causes in my district. After some discussion, during a year when the Ashtabula County satellite was seeking funds to build a new health sciences building, Kent State hit upon the idea that they might prioritize that wish list and said simply that their number one ask was the new building. It got done.

Additionally, because there are a number of organizations that represent nurses and the issues they care about, it is not uncommon to get a different wish list from the same profession. It is not a problem when the issue is specific to the group, but when it is under the "nurse umbrella," coordination among nursing advocates on "the most important issue" would help. When the nurse anesthetists were having a dustup with the anesthesiologists a few years ago about who could, and under what circumstances, provide anesthesia services, it was perfectly understandable that I would hear from that group on that issue. Conversely, when the issue is more global in reach and not confined to a specialty, it is not uncommon to receive a number of different answers regarding the number one issue nurses want addressed. Everyone understands the differences that may exist among different groups that advocate for nurses. However, when there is no cohesive ask for relief on the number one issue, nurses run the risk of the example I used with Kent State. When I cannot figure out which issue is most important to nurses or am getting different views from nurses on how to address it, it does not take a lot of imagination to figure out why it does not get fixed. Realizing that nurses are not homogenized on all issues, there are still matters upon which the official nurse perspective would help. As Congress slogged through the Affordable Care Act the last couple of years, I can honestly say that I never completely understood where nurses were on the bill. The high esteem in which the public and I hold nurses provides an excellent opportunity for nurses to have a seat at the table to advance a position. If the profession's position is unsettled or unclear it is a little bit like the empty chair set for Elijah at the Passover Seder.

Before concluding, I do want to tell one more story about lobbying as it relates to the turf war between the anesthesiologists and the nurses. I had taken the nurses side in the dispute, and the anesthesiologists were anxious to change my view. They invited me to the Cleveland Clinic to watch them in action and observe an operation. After I was appropriately gowned and scrubbed, they led me into the patient's room as the final tubes were being inserted for the spinal block. The patient's back was facing me when I walked in, and I dutifully admired the mass of tubing on the betadine-stained skin, doing my best to "ahhh" appropriately. Then the patient turned around, and it turned out I knew him. Not a huge HIPPA (Health Insurance Portability and Accountability Act) moment but stunning nonetheless. I then went into the operating theater, was introduced to the surgeon, and inquired as to what I would be seeing that day. When you are a 50-something male, as I am, the words "prostate surgery" are probably not the most welcome. It did give the chance, however, when I saw the patient at lunch 2 weeks later to observe that I had certainly seen a lot of him lately. Needless to say, the nurses still had my support.

The bottom line is that everyone who is any good at doing her or his job is probably busy most of the time working to do that job better. I have tried not to be too harsh on nurses in how they navigate Capitol Hill, and I firmly believe that the dedication and time constraints of America's nurses make lobbying Congress an afterthought. However, remembering that anything worth doing is worth doing right, it would be useful if some of the observations I have made could be implemented. Nurses are in a unique position to influence policy and public opinion. You will go as far as the effort that you put into the pursuit.

Nursing Leadership: The Symphony Conductor

Johnnie Maier

Commentary
by Joyce J. Fitzpatrick

*In Maier's description, the true leader is the symphony conductor, who creates the **vision** and the **direction** that merges the many sounds into harmony. The outcome is the symphony's performance, one in which the individual instruments are not distinguishable, but rather come together in unison, often in remarkable ways. Nurse leaders would do well to study the orchestra conductor's understanding of his/her work and leadership role.*

The leader who is a "one-man band" cannot ever be as good as each of the members of the group. Sometimes, micromanaging comes naturally to nurses as they have been socialized to take into account all aspects of a person's life in order to help move the person toward health. In reality in clinical practice, the nurse often is the "one-man band," making sure that everything gets done on the patient care unit, and managing a wide array of activities and persons. But this is management, not leadership, and often the best managers do not make good leaders. To refer to another well-known illustration that is often used to distinguish management and leadership: the forest and the trees. The leader must have the vision to see the forest. It is sometimes most difficult to see the forest when you are scrambling among the trees.

> *As a result of his legislative experience in the Ohio House of Representatives, Maier witnessed the contentious discussions among members of sub-groups within the nursing profession. Because of the foresight, the vision, and the direction of a few legislative leaders, the health care professions involved, nurses and others, were able to play their instruments together. For Maier, the most important lesson for a nurse leader is to learn the skills of the symphony conductor—achieving harmony, balance, and an extraordinary performance without making a sound.*

Key focus areas: advocate, balancing, people sensitivity, big picture

> *The great leaders are like the best conductors—they reach beyond the notes to reach the magic in the players.*
>
> — BLAINE LEE

The most important person in the orchestra does not make a sound. The most important person in the orchestra does not try to sit in every section, attempting to play the different instruments. The most important person in the orchestra conducts the various sections and is the leader whose vision and direction creates the final outcome. The conductor is the leader, the maestro who makes sure all the instruments play in harmony, that all of the various elements come together in unison to produce the desired effect: a fantastic performance.

Observing the orchestra conductor is key to understanding how good leadership should work. A conductor cannot try to play each and every instrument during the performance. The instruments are too many, the mechanics in playing them too varied. The successful maestro cannot master every instrument that comprises the whole of the orchestra, producing the requisite harmony, balance, and rich sound all on his own. The successful conductor is not the micromanager. The "one-man band" model is not appropriate, as a good orchestra is only as good as the sum of its parts. This is also true of successful leadership. The micromanager, the leader who tries to be the proverbial one-man band, will never "reach beyond the notes to reach the magic in the players." In essence, he is not a leader at all, and as a result, diminishes the importance and effectiveness of the individual artists, skilled as they are in their specialized craft, which diminishes the sound of the orchestra as a whole.

A good leader, like a good conductor, works with vision and direction to bring all of the pieces together to achieve the desired end result. The maestro cannot conduct if he is too busy trying to play all the instruments for all the musicians.

A leader must combine vision and direction with an understanding of those he seeks to lead. In an orchestra, the conductor understands the role and purpose of the string section, the brass section, the percussion section, and so on. Likewise, a skilled leader can identify when the various pieces come together, the parts that each person must play, and the common direction that must be taken by all involved.

The "big picture" is what a leader must personally understand and be able to convey to all involved. It is often difficult to see the big picture, the desired outcome, or the end result. Each component of the task, each person involved, like each performer in the orchestra, may only see the outcome from his narrow perspective. The cello player is most concerned with how the cello sounds. Indeed, the leader himself needs to be careful to ensure he is not seeing the outcome solely from his own personal perspective.

A leader who is merely task oriented, focused only on the mechanics of a given project, knows that certain things must be done in order to achieve an end result. He sees the end result as only the conclusion of a number of processes. This person will often plow through a project, forcing adherence, but never achieving a true commitment from all involved. An effective leader must strike the right balance between task orientation and people sensitivity. The successful leader figures out not only what that balance should be, but how it can be achieved.

We refer back to the analogy of the orchestra conductor who, in accomplishing his given task, conducting, realizes the importance of each section in the orchestra to a successful performance. Without proper balance, our orchestra will play the music, but the end result will be a performance that is lacking. Our maestro must have the vision to see everything in front of him. A good leader, like an accomplished conductor, makes sure that those responsible for playing the instruments have bought into the vision, made the commitment, and truly understand the desired outcome, that the orchestra will sound great.

Throughout the nearly 10 years that I served as a member of the Ohio House of Representatives, I worked on hundreds of different bills dealing with various matters of public policy. Health care was always an area of particular interest. Health care issues were often contentious, inside the health care community, as well as to the general public.

During my tenure, I was very active with the passage, and was a cosponsor of Ohio's Nurse Practitioners Act and legislation licensing certified registered nurse anesthetists (CRNA). These pieces of legislation, like the many other bills that came before the Ohio House, required strong leadership for passage. The vision for advancing the scope and practice of the nursing profession, our task, had to be reconciled with a variety of interests within the health care community itself to produce the desired reform and deliver needed change. The passage of both the CRNA Act and the Nurse Practitioners Act has resulted in successful, positive changes to the health care system, and has also had the result of enhancing the nursing profession.

Even though the enactment of these bills resulted in such positive outcomes, the discussions leading to their passage were very contentious. This was true even among some in the nursing profession. These bills invoked a charged and contentious debate among the varied allied health professions.

Those leading the efforts for passage of these two landmark pieces of nursing legislation had the daunting task of bringing the various professions of the health care system into a process that would allow them to accept and understand the vision. A number of people in the nursing profession truly believed that they did not become nurses to advocate for legislation, or to become involved politically. They became nurses to help people; attend to the sick, assist those in need, and to administer the care they were trained to provide. In their view, the motivation to enter the nursing profession had nothing to do with professional advocacy and the legislative process.

They needed to be aware that members of other health care professions felt threatened by the nursing profession expanding its scope of practice. Some believed this increase in scope of practice could not be justified as they believed the nurses' training was not sufficient for these enhanced responsibilities. In addition, others in the health care field were concerned that if nurses could be licensed to do more, it would be at the expense of their particular profession. Those concerned with turf-protection issues, those concerned with competency issues, and the "we have always done it this way" crowd had to be convinced that the passage of this legislation, this new vision for nursing was something that all parties could endorse. Today, we see nurses in the operating room, in the doctor's office, and elsewhere practicing as CRNAs and advanced practice nurses (APNs).

We do not give a lot of thought to the effort required to get to where we are today. The health care system is enhanced. As a result, people enjoy good treatment and skilled care. It is important to remember that the reforms we see as common sense today did not come easily.

The leaders in this process had the foresight to enact these changes in the nursing profession. They possessed clear vision and, more important, the ability to impart that vision upon various, and often competing, forces. This was a prime example of balancing task orientation with people sensitivity. The leaders in the Ohio Legislature were the conductors. And, thankfully, the health care professionals played the instruments. Although I cannot speak for all my colleagues, it is probably prudent that legislators, for the most part, are not working in an operating room.

In order for a leader to be, as I term it, "people sensitive," the leader must understand the needs, motivations, and perceptions of those he or she hopes to lead. As mentioned earlier, nurses become nurses with the motivation to do nursing. Directing people from the focus of their craft to professional advocacy requires the person looking to reform public policy, the leader, moving people, willingly, in a purposeful direction. To be successful, one needs to be very cognizant of the individual's needs and concerns. Therefore, people sensitivity is required to move an individual to the leadership/advocacy role.

After leaving the Ohio House of Representatives owing to term limits, I was elected to the position of municipal clerk of court.

This new position, administrative in nature, required me to put together a staff. Most recently, I had the opportunity to promote a staff person I hired to a supervisory position. This individual is an excellent employee, knowledgeable in her job, and takes an appropriate ownership and leadership role within our office. She is truly invested in the positive operation and development of the office.

When she was hired, she was looking for a good job and a stable position. These were purely economic motivations. Although her work ethic and approach are very positive, I do not believe she was originally coming to our office with the same traits she now exhibits. She came to us initially out of necessity. She grew into the position, grew into leadership, and grew into her current supervisory role.

Before we explore what might have caused this individual to move into a strong leadership/ownership role, I pause to reflect upon my own leadership philosophy, forged through my own professional journey. My first supervisory position occurred when I was 22 years old, working in a youth detention facility. I made mistakes, and at the time had very little in the way of resources to guide me. As we all do, I grew in my professional knowledge and abilities. After nearly 40 years of supervision and leadership experience, I have developed a personal philosophy and vision about leadership. I believe that I am a much better leader today than I was earlier in my life.

One of my core beliefs is that people work in order to live. People, by and large, do not live in order to work. This is not to understate the fact that work is an integral and often personally satisfying aspect of our lives. It should be part of a well-balanced life, and not the totality of one's existence.

The staff person I recently promoted had shared with me that one of her lifelong dreams was to be a track coach. This dream of hers was a far stretch from working as a deputy clerk of court. Additionally, working as a track coach was a seasonal type of endeavor that would fall far short of satisfying her family's economic necessities. She soon became aware of an opportunity for a position at a local high school coaching girls track. She did not see how she could pursue this opportunity, because our office was open until 4:30 p.m., and the track practice started at 3:00 p.m. We found a very simple way to accommodate her scheduling needs. She was scheduled to report to work 2 hours early, and became the staff member who would prepare the necessary documents for morning court. This simple accommodation enabled her to fulfill her coaching dreams. Now, her job with the court was enabling her to more fully live her life and pursue her other goals. People work in order to live. The effect of this change is that her personal fulfillment has resulted in an individual developing a deep sense of loyalty, leadership, and ownership within our office.

This is a tale of "people sensitivity," in which someone was able to advance up Abraham Maslow's famous "hierarchy of needs." Because our staff person's economic needs were addressed, she could live more fully, "move up the pyramid," and enjoy more intrinsically satisfying pursuits. Her increased self-esteem, confidence, and achievement spilled over to her work, and as a result, her leadership role developed more fully.

To draw a parallel to professional nursing advocacy, it is important that the motivation that drew an individual to the field of nursing can be mustered to see the bigger picture. As one's economic needs are met through performing one's craft, one's desire to care for others can be enhanced through professional advocacy. Advocacy work improves the profession, thereby instilling someone with esteem, confidence, and the achievement that comes from effecting positive change. Helping to care for others and professional advocacy that improves the quality of care for others achieves the same goal, helping others.

Another personal example of helping someone meet his own needs, while also simultaneously fulfilling the organization's needs, occurred when I was the manager of the staff for a number of group homes. I had put together an initial staff schedule. When I distributed the schedule, one of the staff members looked at it, handed it back to me, and stated that because of the schedule, he could no longer work at the group home. The problem was that I had scheduled the individual to work on a Thursday afternoon, which was the one day of the week that he needed to pick his daughter up from elementary school. Work had now become a major interference with his parental requirements, the responsibility to his daughter. This situation could have been resolved in a number of ways in which the outcome would have been less than positive. I chose to make the necessary accommodation, having empathy for his situation, understanding that enabling this staff member to fulfill his obligations to his young daughter was critical. This individual became my most trusted employee, working above and beyond the call of duty, and becoming a strong advocate for the group-home residents.

Returning once more to our orchestra analogy, in this case, the conductor recognized that the violin player did not have a stand for his sheet music. Without the stand, the violinist could not play. With the music stand the violinist could play wonderfully. The conductor, by providing the stand to hold the music, never produced a musical note, yet created the environment for it to occur. With his daughter's situation resolved, the group home staff member could pursue his work, at which he was quite good.

These analogies, these stories, I hope, lead to the realization that leaders need to create the environment, indeed the capacity, for others to become leaders as well. The path to leadership, and, following in that vein, the path to professional advocacy, is created by those in leadership.

For nursing to keep pace with changing health care needs, nursing must change also. Change is the one constant, it is inevitable. As such, the leaders in the profession, those with vision, our "change agents" must be the ones who enable and grow the next generation of leaders. For individuals to assume the professional advocacy role, it must be understood that this role, which is often perceived to be very different from the role of the practitioner, is indeed similar. The efforts of the advocate may achieve goals comparable to those of the practitioner, often on a larger scale.

In developing individuals as leaders and as advocates, it is necessary to understand how an individual reaches this stage. It is not through the mentoring, or the example of the micromanager, the so-called one-man band. It is by learning why a skilled maestro, our orchestra conductor, achieves harmony, balance, and an extraordinary performance as the person who, without making a sound, or playing an instrument, is the most important person in the orchestra.

Factoring the role of the leader with the development of true leadership is critical to a better understanding of the constant need to further develop advocacy within the profession. The end result of the advocate and of the practitioner is the same: seeking a better way to serve and to heal the sick.

14

Nursing Leadership: As It Should Be

Shawn D. Mathis

Commentary
by Joyce J. Fitzpatrick

*A*ccording to Mathis, leadership is always defined
by the leader's character. Although talent and
skills are important, Mathis underlines the following
core competences for leadership: vigilance, connection,
humility, competence, drive, and sacrifice. Mathis
identifies the true leaders in health care as the nurses
on the front lines, the nurses who "share our pain." He
believes that nurses must be empowered to make the
world a better place. Nurse leaders today would agree
with Mathis; indeed, much of the current emphasis
within health care organizations from the nurse leaders'
perspective is the empowerment of nurses at all levels.

    *Mathis argues that the health care industry has
largely ignored nurses, and the profession has not been
given proper respect, support, or attention. But, importantly, for purposes of understanding the role of the nurse
leader, Mathis rightfully places some of the responsibility
with nurse leaders within the health care industry. He
clearly defines core characteristics that are needed for leadership, and challenges nurses to develop these components
within their work to effect change in health care. His goal is
to be the catalyst for change for nurses, and to change the
health care landscape so that the nurses' voices can be heard.*

Key focus areas: core characteristics (vigilance, connection, humble, competent, drive, sacrifice), passionate, influence, relationships, position of service

Mary clutched her favorite teddy bear. "Sammy go too?" Mary asked.

"No, honey," her mom gently said.

"Sammy go too!" Mary insisted.

"No, Sammy can't go with you because he might be in the doctor's way," Mary's dad responded.

"Sammy go too!" Mary screamed as she started to cry.

Mary's parents were visibly upset about the exchange. For 10 minutes, they had been trying, unsuccessfully, to get Mary to give them her teddy bear so she could be wheeled into the surgery preparation room. It was tough enough to think about their baby going "under the knife" but to "fight" with her before it happened was almost unbearable.

"Juwee," Mary sobbed.

Mary's parents turned to see the nurse who had been working with Mary during her stay in the hospital.

"What's wrong?" Julie asked as she approached Mary.

"Sammy go too?"

Julie smiled. "Are you worried about Sammy?"

Mary nodded her head.

"I tell you what, Mary, why don't you let your mom and dad take care of Sammy for you while you go with the doctor? I promise they will take good care of him. And I will check on him just like I've been checking on you. Okay?"

"Okay, Juwee," was Mary's simple response.

Mary's parents were astonished and her mom followed Julie to the hallway and asked, "How did you do that?"

"I've been watching Mary play with Sammy for the last few days, and I just figured her real concern was whether he would be taken care of while she was in surgery," Julie explained.

Mary's mom smiled, hugged Julie, and stepped back into the room to spend a few precious moments with her daughter.

It's a simple story. So simple, in fact, that some will read it and wonder why I chose to include it in a book related to nursing leadership.

The answer is as simple as the story. To me, the story reveals key characteristics of leadership. Characteristics that must be mined, developed, and rewarded. Characteristics that should be present in any individual who desires to be a leader. Characteristics that must be found in those who would be leaders in nursing.

Before I explain what the story reveals to me, perhaps a little background is in order. I am a businessman. I have successfully started, led, and sold several companies. I have hired and fired many employees. I have negotiated with, worked alongside, and battled "stalwarts" in industry, I know the difference between visionary leadership enacted and lame duck leadership that simply creates complexity. I have seen great leaders, and I have seen abysmal leaders. It is my goal and mission to be an effective, positive leader.

What have I discovered as a scholar of leadership, both historically and present day? Leadership is always defined by a leader's character.

Talent alone does not cut it. No matter how talented you are in budget development and strategic planning, if the core of your character is not what it should be, you will turn around and find that no one is following you, or if they are, they are there for the wrong reasons.

Skills alone do not cut it. It does not matter how skilled you are in presentations or decision making, if the core of your character is not worth following, your leadership journey will more closely resemble a solitary walk, or worse a tyrannical power.

Do not get me wrong. Talent and skills are important, but any good manager can display both talent and skill, and not rise to the level of a leader. Because you cannot be a leader without the ability to inspire others and lead them, and you will not have followers without the right core values displayed in your character on a day in, day out basis.

What are the right core characteristics for leadership? I think it boils down to the following concepts: vigilance, connection, humility, competence, drive, and sacrifice.

Leaders are vigilant. They are aware of everything that is happening around them. They pay attention to industry trends. They understand the needs of their customers. They listen to their employees. Their focus is neither outside nor inside their company but a balanced combination of both. They are standing in the hallway to hear the cries of a little girl because they are ever-watchful of those they lead.

Leaders are connected. They observe. They ask questions. They listen. They build relationships. They engage the heart and the mind. They are able to determine that a little girl needs her teddy bear to be cared for because they are "checked in" with their followers. Details matter for leaders, and they are careful to lead even in the details of knowing and interacting in details important to their people.

Leaders are humble. They have ambition, but it is not related to their personal achievements. Their ambition is turned toward their company, their colleagues, and their followers. They are willing to talk about a little girl's teddy bear as if it is real because positive end results are not about their "dignity," they are about the team.

Leaders are competent. They know their stuff. They even know the things they do not know. They surround themselves with people who know their stuff too. And they encourage those people to be competent in their roles. They are willing to be part of the supporting cast—especially when it means setting up a little girl's parents as heroes to her and her teddy bear. Leaders know when to use their influence and, more important, they know when influence can best be used for good.

Leaders have drive. They are passionate about their work. They care about results. They cannot wait to get up and get on the job every day. They do not shy away from a challenge. They are willing to deal with the difficult situations. They do the things we cannot imagine doing. And the tasks can be large or small—even a little girl's cries over a teddy bear drive them to excellence.

Leaders sacrifice. They embrace the enormous responsibilities that come with leadership. They give up personal aspirations to meet the needs of their followers. They take the bad shifts and tough wards. They help a frightened little girl while their own daughter rides the bus to school.

The leaders I respect are individuals who embody these characteristics. And they pass the ultimate test of leadership—they influence people, and by their actions people are inspired and drawn to act on their influence.

In the health care industry, most of these leaders are not in the C-suite, wearing Brooks Brother's suits and handing out business cards with fancy titles. The true leaders of the health care industry are on the front lines of health care delivery, wearing stained scrubs, and hearing their names called 24 hours a day, 365 days a year. Ask their former patients about a hospital stay and listen to what the patients discuss. They may give a couple of seconds to the doctor who saw them, but the majority of their conversations will turn to their relationships with nurses. And those interactions will dictate whether their hospital experience was good or difficult. That is true influence, and the nurse's ability to truly affect a patient's experience is leadership!

Unfortunately, the health care industry has largely failed to recognize its true front-line influencers. It has failed at upholding and listening to the very voices that not only carry out chart orders but very often spend the most time with the clients they serve. Take a closer look at the C-suite in the health care industry. They are "experts" in strategic planning, budgeting, cost control, and nurse acquisition, but they have no idea how to lead. In many instances, those "leaders" are tacticians who have not served a single patient in their careers. They have not been in the personal position of service to a single human interaction in their career. How can they lead an industry that involves patient care when they have never cared for a patient? They lack a fundamental characteristic of leadership—they are not connected to the experience the nurse industry experiences every day—the responsibility of caring, of nurturing, and of providing the best practices in health care every day to the client—the patients.

In the rare situations in which "working" nurses are appointed to C-suite positions, the very characteristics that made them leaders on the floor are quickly drained out of them as they are asked to focus their attention on organizational concerns rather than patient care. The C-suite's focus on "organizational concerns" is particularly shortsighted because it fails to address the needs of its front-line workers. The health care industry has flatly ignored nurses in many instances. For years, the nursing profession has not been given proper respect, support, or attention. For too long, the C-suite has scrutinized nurse care as a line item instead of recognizing its critical role in the delivery of health care.

Simply put, the nurse or health industry has not taken care of its nurses.

It is a deplorable situation because those same nurses take care of us in our greatest times of joy, sadness, pain, and physical need. It is a monumental failure of nurse industry "leadership" because organizational strength is often measured by how an organization treats its people. And nurses are crying out that our health care organizations are lacking, they know what they are talking about, and their voices deserve to be heard. It is a tragic result for our patients because each day we fail to listen to our front-line warriors in the fight for quality patient care, we waste lives.

In my experience, businesses are successful when their products remain true to their original purposes. In health care, the product's purpose is nurture of and care for patients. We cannot take our eyes off the goal—the health care industry's purpose is to relieve pain and suffering. I do not know when everyone else was introduced to the pain and suffering in our world, but my introduction came when I was 5 years old when my cancer-stricken mom asked for water.

I heard my mom's voice. I knew I should go see what she wanted, but I was not sure what to expect. She had been in the hospital a lot and she looked different from the mom I was used to seeing. She was sort of gray. She did not have much hair. She vomited. She cried. She seemed really weak. She just wasn't her. And, to be honest, it scared me a little. My dad said I should help her as much as I could, so I walked into the living room. In a hard-to-understand and muffled utterance my Mom said, "Water."

I turned, headed toward the kitchen, found a cup, turned on the tap, placed the cup under it, got the water, went back to the living room, and handed the drink to her.

"Help?"

At first, I wasn't sure what she meant. But as she touched her lips, I started to understand. Her lips were swollen and stuck together and she could not get them apart to drink the water, so I did my best to open them and put the cup to her mouth. She groaned a bit, but she was finally able to take a sip of the water.

"Thank you."

My mom beat cancer. But I haven't been able to shake that image of pain and suffering viewed from the eyes of her 5-year- old son.

It is a painful perspective, but one that enlightens my desire for every global citizen to have access to men and women who will take care of them during his or her most painful experiences.

Consider Henri Nouwen's words, "When we honestly ask ourselves which person in our lives means the most to us, we often find that it is those who, instead of giving advice, solutions, or cures, have chosen rather to share our pain and touch our wounds with a warm and tender hand."

I cannot read that passage without thinking about the calling and leadership of nurses.

Nurses understand that not every patient will beat cancer or recover from the wounds of the car accident or cheat death one more time through an emergency heart surgery. Nurses know some people will lose the fight and their life.

Despite this knowledge, men and women choose to become nurses to "share our pain" and "touch our wounds" with their "warm and tender" hands.

In a world marked by pain and suffering, that desire means everything. And their influence makes nurses the true leaders of the health care industry.

If we are to meet the physical and spiritual needs of the world's citizens, we must empower our nurses. We must embrace the principle that nursing is personal, and the real art and power of nursing is the one-on-one nurse–patient relationship. We must acknowledge the failures of our current system. We must change the leadership status quo. We must embrace the expansion of our nurses' influence throughout our health care organizations.

Does this mean more nurses should be appointed to C-suite positions? That would not hurt, but I am not talking about mere changes of position or title. Remember, leadership is about influence, not position.

I am asking for an upside-down approach to leadership in the health care industry. The only way we will address our world's health care needs is if the collective voice of nurses rules the day in organizational decision making. We must capture the character of our nurses—their vigilance, connection, humility, competence, drive, and sacrifice—and demonstrate the same leadership throughout our health care organizations. And we must embrace the visionary force guiding these characteristics in our nurses—deep, meaningful, personalized patient care.

We have endured decades of other approaches to leadership in the health care industry, and the results are dismal at best. High burnout and turnover rates among nurses plague us as we watch our worldwide population age and anticipate its growing health care needs. Nurse faculty shortages lead to fewer and fewer nursing students among the next generation of nurses. Those who graduate from nursing school are routinely rejected by the conventional wisdom of the C-suite as lacking enough experience to hire. Meanwhile, pain and suffering continues in every part of our globe, and there are not enough nurses to share the pain and touch the wounds.

It is time for the health care industry to recognize what Mary did—Julie is a leader worth following. And if our patients—who are the clients in our health care industry—recognize nurses as leaders, does it not make sense that we should too?

15

Nursing Leadership: Pushing Ohio Slowly Forward

Joan Mazzolini

Commentary
by Joyce J. Fitzpatrick

*M*azzolini suggests that nurse leaders in Ohio need to step up their game and move more quickly at the political and policy development levels to effect changes in health care. The stories she recounts are all too familiar, when as early as 1994 changes were implemented to recognize the value of advanced practice nurses in delivering care to underserved populations. The results were incremental, and some of the desired changes are only now being addressed by the state legislators, more than 18 years since the initial discussions were brought forward by a small group of nurse leaders.

Maximizing resources for the attainment of societal goals is an important goal for nurse leaders, in any locale. Mazzolini believes that nurses have missed the mark in telling their story to the public. Even though nurses are consistently identified as the most trusted health professionals and nurse leaders often tout this fact, most people have very little understanding of the roles that nurses play or could play in health care delivery. And the legislators often do not understand the barriers that restrict nursing practice, or are slow to address these barriers.

Nurses struggle with getting the work out, and, according to Mazzolini, nurses are not using the resources

> *available to them, for example, social media and the Internet. Thus, the nurse leaders are characterized as too patient to make a difference, too timid to make the necessary changes and let their voices be heard. Too often the nurse leaders are under the radar, rather than being driving forces for change. We have learned this lesson many times over in Ohio; we have all been there on the sidelines. Perhaps following Mazzolini's advice, it is time for a change, for an active, direct confrontation of the health care issues both at the state and at the national levels.*

Key focus areas: patient, persevere, harness the power, maximizing resources, collective effort

When I moved back to Cleveland to take a reporting job at the *Plain Dealer* in late 1991, I expected my home state to be on the cutting edge of medical care and health policy compared with Alabama, where I happily covered the business of health and public health for nearly 4 years while a reporter at the now defunct *Birmingham Post-Herald*.

I had graduated from The Ohio State University with a business degree; my major was finance, but I had decided that was not for me. After working for a couple of years, I moved to Alaska and spent a little more than a year living in Anchorage, going to school part time, working and traveling the state.

I left Alaska to go to graduate school at Northwestern University's Medill School of Journalism, and after the program took the job in Birmingham. Although smaller in size, Birmingham has a lot of similarities to Cleveland, including a history of manufacturing steel, and a large medical community with a medical school; a university hospital; a veterans hospital; and several hospital competitors, including a for-profit hospital in the region.

Alabama, which was considerably poorer than Ohio at the time, had innovative public health leaders pushing to ensure the poor and uninsured had access to quality care.

So when I moved back to Cleveland I was surprised. There were several areas in which Ohio was, to put it politely, behind compared with Alabama and the United States.

And clearly one of those arenas was in the appreciation and understanding of the roles nurses could and should play in ensuring medical care—especially in physician-shortage areas such as inner-city neighborhoods and rural communities.

As I looked into the issue of doctor shortages, the debate—some would say controversy—over not allowing nurse practitioners the ability to practice somewhat independently became crystallized. It was something that had been tackled in a majority of the states, but in Ohio, with a large number of medical schools but not a single school of public health (at that time), issues between doctors and nurses were more complicated. And leadership from the Ohio Department of Health, which traditionally had physicians' directors with no expertise in public health, was not forthcoming. Nurses, collectively, have been patiently pursuing a course of action that has them butting against the medical establishment not for financial gain but specifically because patients would benefit.

Although the traditional definition of leadership often highlights a singular effort of one person directing, guiding, leading—a more expanded definition includes themes such as what Alan Keith of Genentech said of leadership: "creating ways for people to contribute to making something extraordinary happen."

Or as professor of leadership Ken "SKC" Ogbonnia, who defines leadership as, "the ability to successfully integrate and maximize available resources within the internal and external environment for the attainment of organizational or societal goals." (Pascoe, 2011).

It is that definition—maximizing resources for the attainment of society's goals—that I believe has propelled Ohio's nurses forward. Although "leaders" have changed in the movement, the collective effort to get Ohio laws rewritten has been consistent.

However, I believe nurses, who are often beloved by patients, have somehow missed the mark in the collective telling of their story. I believe that if that area was markedly improved, Ohioans would push our timid, wayward, and off-the-mark legislature to move forward on issues that other states have passed us by on that seem to drag on for years, maybe decades, in Ohio.

In 1993, when I was reporting on a story about nurse practitioners getting some freedom, the feeling that momentum was behind the nurses' efforts was palpable. Ultimately, though, it would take years for real results.

My story (Mazzolini, 1994) ran in early January of 1994. These were the first few paragraphs to the front-page story:

"An empty bank building in Cleveland is the unlikely site for the start of health care reform.

"When the renovation of the old Society Bank building on Buckeye Rd. is completed in late March, the result will be a health care center unique to Greater Cleveland and the nation—but not for long. The bank soon will be a primary care and birthing center run by nurses."

Later in the story I got to the crux of the issue:

"In Ohio, primary care providers are needed now. Fifty-two of the state's 88 counties, including Cuyahoga, where there is a nationally recognized medical school and an excess of hospitals, are federally designated as medically underserved.

"To fill these health care gaps caused by the shortage of primary care physicians, schools of nursing at CWRU [Case Western Reserve University] and in other parts of the country are giving nurses more advanced training. The movement started before the Clinton push for health reform. But it fits the goals of that effort.

"'We're just ahead of the change,' said Joyce J. Fitzpatrick, dean of the Frances Payne Bolton School of Nursing at CWRU.

"The change is the expanded role of nurse practitioners to provide basic care, such as physical or prenatal exams, immunizations, and prescribing high blood pressure medications.

"The Cleveland nursing center is one of three pilot programs being developed in Ohio under state legislation passed last year. The others are at Wright State University in Dayton and in Cincinnati. A similar pilot program is being discussed in Columbus. For now, the Cleveland center will be the only one that does both primary care and baby delivery."

The story touched on the issue that state lawmakers needed to pass legislation to give the advanced practice nurses (APNs) in Ohio something more than 40 states had already done—the ability to write prescriptions.

"Nurse practitioners had worked for years to pass such legislation in Ohio, but doctor groups worked to prohibit it. The Ohio Medical Association's position is that nurse practitioners are competent care-givers, but they need the supervision of physicians and shouldn't have the ability to write prescriptions.

"'We have a hard enough time making sure our doctors prescribe correctly,' said Dr. Walter Reiling Jr., president of the Ohio Medical Association.

"Legislation also was needed to officially recognize nurse practitioners and nurse midwives in Ohio, giving them 'title recognition' and thus the ability to bill an insurance company or Medicaid for their services. That legislation also passed last year."

That nursing center did not last. And I would like to say that a tremendous amount had changed over the past 17 years in Ohio in terms of the lawmakers' attitudes on nursing, but I would be wrong.

Instead, it has been the patience of Ohio's nursing community that has stood out and their persistence to push forward an agenda to help patients not with any one person getting the credit. But again, I would be remiss if I did not say that these issues important to nurses often get lost in the state capital and in the minds of the average Ohio resident.

The old saying "the more things change, the more they stay the same" comes to mind. After I moved to other beats, I watched the reporters covering the business of health and medicine in Ohio and saw the same stories, same issues, same problems cycle through again and again.

And when I was asked to cover the medical/health beat for a short while, it was a déjà vu story that I did in December of 2008.

The story was about "doctor extenders," including nurse practitioners and physician assistants, who earn much less than physicians but are desperately needed to fill a hole in the nation's preventive and primary care positions.

I noted that it was not until the year 2000 when Ohio lawmakers finally passed a law to allow advanced practice nurses to prescribe drugs. Ohio, despite having numerous health shortage areas, was the last state in the country.

In late 2008, the issue was expanding the rules to let nurse practitioners prescribe Schedule II medications, which include narcotics. The law then only allowed them to prescribe a 1-day supply of pain medications to a terminally ill patient, and only if a doctor wrote the original prescription.

Again Ohio was behind, with about 31 other states allowing APNs to prescribe Schedule II drugs without restrictions. And Ohio, unlike many other states, also requires nurse practitioners to work collaboratively with a supervisory doctor.

Jacalyn Golden, a nurse practitioner and at the time the legislative chairwoman for the state association, noted, "Why can we do it for 24 hours, but why not 48, or a week?"

The Ohio State Medical Association's senior director for government affairs, said, "We don't want to be blurring the lines between the practice of medicine and the practice of nursing."

Again, the issue arose of nurses stepping in to fill the acute need of patients in shortage areas, where there are not just shortages of primary care doctors but specialists as well.

I left the reporting profession almost a year and a half ago. But the goal of nurse practitioners prescribing Schedule II drugs has only recently passed in the state legislature.

Doing a quick check on the Ohio Nurses Association website, I saw familiar themes: nurses working to get the recognition that they are qualified "providers of health care services including prescriptive services."

The association is also working to enable consumers to get "direct access . . . to services of registered nurses" and getting "direct reimbursement to nurses in advanced practice roles."

A story last year in the *Dayton Daily News* (Bishoff, 2011) again brought up the issue of passing legislation to allow APNs to prescribe Schedule II drugs.

"Nurses frame the issue in terms of providing better access to primary care for patients, while doctors cite concerns about patient safety," the story said.

"Intensifying the debate in recent months are two Ohio bills— one that would expand APNs' ability to prescribe certain medications, and another that would create pilot programs to test a kind of family medicine that incentivizes preventive health care."

The issues covered in the story had exactly the same themes as the story I did back in 1994. My question or challenge to Ohio nurses is, why have they not used the tools that did not exist in 1994— basically the Internet and now other forms of communication— to help drive their agenda? When I did a search to see the stories written in the past year and a half on these and other nursing issues, I found very few. And although part of the blame goes to the newspaper industry and the seeming lack of direction in covering important stories as well as little interest in public health and public issues, some of the blame must be laid on Ohio's nursing leaders, as well. This may be the area where individual leaders—the current and past deans of Ohio's various nursing schools and others—must come out to speak strongly on these issues.

Although I have touted the leadership of nurses in being able to be patient and persevere while the issues have dragged out, I must also criticize that patience and the inability to harness the Internet, blogs, and so on (I am not a fan of Twitter except in the case of independence movements) to get more information out on these issues and use the power of the public to help move Ohio forward.

I searched for information, stories, and so on on the pilot projects for a concept called patient-centered medical homes. The few items I could find indicated that the Ohio House and Senate had approved the bill and that Gov. Strickland signed it to allow 44 pilot programs to be established, with four set aside for advanced practice nurses.

So, although it seems they are being established, not much beyond the websites of associations or colleges has much information. The *Columbus Dispatch* did a short story on doctor-led centers and mentioned that there would be APN centers.

My new job is as communications officer (communications director if I did not work for a foundation where the term *officer* is the preferred term) for the Sisters of Charity Foundation of Cleveland. The foundation's endowment came from the sale of half of St. Vincent Charity Hospital (now medical center) to a for-profit hospital chain. The Sisters of Charity of St. Augustine resold that half later to University Hospitals and in the last few years bought the half back.

And although the foundation is not run by nuns, their culture of doing their work without any real acknowledgment or fame is definitely felt and in some ways permeates the work of the foundation.

Last year I attended the Cleveland showing of "Women and Spirit: Catholic Sisters in America," which started at the Smithsonian and is touring the country. I bring this up because one of the exhibits highlighted the Sister and her religious order that started what we now refer to as the Mayo Clinic.

Unfortunately, I cannot remember the name of the Sister who was instrumental in its founding. "Histories" mention the nuns of St. Francis as being instrumental in building the first hospital of the Mayo Clinic.

William Mayo immigrated to Minnesota and became a doctor. His two sons followed in his footsteps. So although the name Mayo is now synonymous with exceptional hospital care, the Sister (who was likely a public health nurse) and her order, who were instrumental in its inception, are relegated to the footnotes of history.

My retelling of this story is obvious. Although I believe the best leaders are often not tooting their own horns, their stories get out. And they have to if the change of direction they hope to effect gets traction and builds. Otherwise, how would we know they were leaders?

Nurses in Ohio and the issues important to them have been under the radar for too long. I understand that the culture of nursing, the training, and maybe the leadership have been to put the patient first, which is honorable. But to effect the change nurses hope and long for in Ohio, the culture must evolve.

I wonder whether careers that are by majority female headed, such as nursing, suffer from a similar ailment that the salaries of the majority of "female" careers suffer from. Everyone talks of the importance of these careers yet the workers are often underpaid and taken for granted.

The political attack on public school teachers—with the term *public* somehow turned into a dirty word—may be a cautionary tale but also a learning tool for nurses moving into the public forefront.

Although a united front and the leaders who have slowly moved Ohio nursing issues forward have worked, the gains have been painstakingly slow.

Either the united front and the behind-the-scenes leaders need to move to the forefront or others need to step forward to be the "face" for the issues. Studies show that nursing care at hospitals is more highly regarded and drives patient decisions more than doctor care.

Ohio nurses need to harness that power into the future. Not to put any pressure on you, but the American health care system is at stake.

REFERENCES

Bischoff, L. A. (2010, March 6). Doctors, nurses battle over roles in health care. *Dayton Daily News*. Retrieved from http://www.daytondaily news.com/news/news/state-regional/doctors-nurses-battle-over-roles-in-health-care-1/nM9q7/

Mazzolini, J. (1994, January 3). At new health center, doctor won't be in, but nurse will. *Cleveland Plain Dealer*.

Pascoe, R. R. (2011). *The Uncompromising Leader*. Maitland, FL: Xulon Press.

16

Perspectives on Nursing Leadership: From a Physician Chief Executive Officer

David C. Pate

Commentary
by Joyce J. Fitzpatrick

*P*ate learned about nurses as leaders from an early experience as a volunteer in a busy surgical intensive care unit (SICU). This early experience shaped his views as a physician. Before entering medical school, Pate understood that nurses had an extremely important leadership role to play in patient care. Based on Pate's experience, we might want to expose premedical students to nursing, so that the stereotypes are eliminated before new cultural patterns are learned. The professional status imbalance between medicine and nursing is often learned in medical and nursing education, and certainly often is dominant in the clinical arenas. Thus, physicians and nurses often have to unlearn their stereotypic views. Better that we design ways to avoid learning the stereotypes so as to save time in the unlearning process.

Pate further elaborates his value for front-line nurses as leaders in the Magnet-designated hospitals in which he has worked. In fact, he so values the Magnet principles and culture that he would have refused the chief executive officer (CEO) position that he currently holds if the hospital was not a Magnet hospital. This is an important statement for all nurse leaders and health care executives to hear.

> *One of Pate's most important messages is the potential for nursing leadership in health care delivery in the future. It is important for nurses to capture the opportunities in the changes that will inevitably take place with the needs for patient- and family-centered care. Pate believes that nurse leaders are prepared for the challenges ahead.*

Key focus areas: shared governance, team-based care, culture, advanced education, pursuit of excellence

To understand my views on nursing leadership, it is appropriate to explain my views on nursing and how they developed. I knew from a very young age that I wanted to be a doctor. I did not know any nurses growing up to shape my views on nursing. Many of my impressions were shaped by television shows that at that time, with few exceptions, portrayed nurses as minor characters relative to the physicians and never revealed the full nature and role of nursing in patient care.

MY INTRODUCTION TO NURSING

In college, I decided to volunteer at a medical center hospital to learn more about my chosen career, in specific, and health care, in general. I was assigned to the SICU at a Level I trauma center. I had no idea at the time what a profound experience this would be.

I was very intimidated, to say the least. I had never seen patients so ill. I was overwhelmed by the complex machines, the vast number of tubes and lines, and the never-ending alarms that rotated from one side of the room to another.

Unlike most of the television shows I had seen (late 1960s and early 1970s), which seemed to portray a relaxed and unhurried atmosphere in which nurses typically were taking vital signs or administering a shot, I saw that nurses were always busy caring for their patients, administering medications, suctioning endotracheal tubes, draining and measuring catheters and tubes, drawing blood for tests, responding to alarms, repositioning their patients, examining and evaluating their patients, discussing the care of their patients with physicians and other care givers, talking to families and those very few patients who could hear and understand (and probably more impactful to me, talking to those patients who could not). I was impressed by how much knowledge nurses had and how they cared for their patients.

I learned many things. First of all, it quickly came into perspective for me that although the physicians rounded through the unit and then were gone, the nurses were there around the clock. Nurses were often the first to pick up on a sign of early distress or deterioration. I realized that families often asked the nurses questions that they did not feel comfortable asking the doctor or when they did not understand the answer given by the doctor.

I appreciated that the nurses spent so much time in explaining things to me. It seemed that in appreciation for the time I gave as a volunteer and the help I provided in lifting, bathing, and weighing patients, they were giving me knowledge and experiences that would shape my views of nursing and my later practice of medicine forever.

The additional benefit of my volunteer experience was that I would meet my future wife in the SICU. She was one of the most knowledgeable and skilled nurses of the many outstanding nurses I met. She taught me to read electrocardiograms (EKGs) and interpret laboratory tests, and she taught me to see patients through the eyes of a nurse. She also taught me to pick up after myself and not to leave a mess at the bedside after performing a procedure on a patient, lessons that would endear me to the nurses I worked with as a physician.

RESIDENCY

The experiences I had as a volunteer and the exposure I had to nursing would affect my practice as a physician starting in my internal medicine residency. I excelled in my residency training and because of this, was selected to serve in the prestigious position of chief resident at the end of my training. I attribute much of this success to nurses. I had an advantage over many of my fellow trainees—I knew that the nurses could pick up on subtleties in my patients that I might very well miss. I listened to the nurses when a lot of my fellow residents ignored them and did not realize how nurses would help them provide better care to their patients. More than once, a nurse kept me from making a mistake. I also knew that in the middle of the night, when I was dealing with a critically ill patient, the nurses could often lead me to the correct treatment for a complex patient.

NURSING LEADERSHIP—MY VIEWS AND PERSPECTIVES AS A PHYSICIAN EXECUTIVE

The Chief Nursing Officer as an Executive

When I first became a CEO of a large, tertiary care, teaching hospital just down the street from the hospital I volunteered at, I put together my team of executives—two nurses (a vice president and chief nursing officer [CNO] and a vice president over our cardiovascular and surgical services), a microbiologist (vice president over accreditation, safety, and the laboratory), and a nonclinician vice president over radiology, emergency management and support services. I explained that each executive was an executive over the entire hospital first, and over his or her portfolio second. Each executive had the right to go into any area of the hospital and ask any questions. The CNO was an integral part of the team— expected to be able to explain the vision, inspire the employees to achieve our goals, demonstrate accountability, participate in setting the strategies, and engage in our team meetings whether the subject involved patient care or not.

Magnet as a Culture

I was very proud that our hospital was one of the first Magnet hospitals in Texas and that we were redesignated each time thereafter. I was committed to shared governance because I knew how important it was to have the perspectives of front-line nurses in making decisions about patient care. I was committed to advanced education and training for nurses because it contributed to better patient care, and I realized how much of the quality of care provided in hospitals is due to nursing assessments and interventions. Furthermore, I saw Magnet as a culture in our hospital to be closely guarded—the continuous pursuit of excellence in nursing and patient care. When I was first contacted about an opportunity to lead the health system I currently serve, the first thing I did was to go online to ensure that the flagship hospital was a Magnet-designated hospital—it was. I honestly would not have engaged in the search process if it was not.

I believe that culture starts at the top. The commitment to excellence, quality, safety, nursing research, advanced practice, staff development, employee engagement, nursing and patient education, and evidence-based practice started with me and my entire executive team and was in evidence every day and in every decision made by my CNO.

Physician–Nurse Relationships

I was privileged to work with an outstanding medical staff. That medical staff recognized that their patients received amazing care because of the outstanding nurses we had. One of the things that helped to retain these outstanding nurses was their desire to be part of a team, to be recognized for their contributions to the team and to patient care, and their desire to learn from physicians. Because so many of our physicians understood this, we had high retention and engagement from our nurses. Together with the medical staff, we set out the expectation that all interactions with employees were to be professional, appropriate, and respectful.

However, on occasion, we were confronted with a disruptive physician. I decided from day one that no physician, no matter how much business she or he brought to our hospital, was worth losing the culture we had worked so hard to maintain. No physician could be excused from treating nurses professionally, appropriately, and respectfully in each and every interaction. Each time an incident occurred, the chief of staff, my Vice President of Medical Affairs, and I intervened to ensure that each nurse felt supported and that we were walking the talk.

THE NURSE LEADER OF THE FUTURE

Just as health care is preparing to go through the biggest change in nearly 50 years, so too, the role of the CNO/nurse executive will change dramatically. The CNO/nurse executive will be critical in redesigning the health care delivery system of the future.

What will change? Everything! First of all, the very care management model must change. It is too fragmented, too inconvenient, too ineffective, and too physician centered. What will the new care management model look like? The reimbursement system must eventually change from fee-for-service to payment for value. When this happens, physicians will no longer be rewarded for personally performed services, but rather for obtaining better outcomes (improved indicators of health/disease management and lower total cost of care) for a panel of patients. This will be the change that will be needed to help move toward team-based care in the outpatient/ambulatory arena. This will mean that physicians will now utilize physician assistants and advanced practice nurses in the management of their patients. Once this happens, patients with chronic medical diseases can be actively managed in between office visits, decreasing the current fragmentation that characterizes our model of care. The CNO/nurse executive will be critical in the creation and implementation of this new care model.

The above changes to the care model are inevitable. However, those health systems that want to be the best will further adapt the care model to be patient centered and family centered. This is another area for leadership from nursing and quite a number of other disciplines. It starts with looking at everything we do from the standpoint of the patient and those who provide the support system for the patient, in both the inpatient and outpatient settings. For example, how effective is our patient education? For the patient who has been admitted to the hospital, are we really effective in educating the patient when he or she is ill, on sedating medications, and sleep deprived? In the physician's office, how much of the information we provide patients will actually be understood and retained? We need to utilize technology and develop education that can be listened to/viewed at home and that has a stop and replay function. We need content that can be shared with all caregivers and that can be forwarded to a family member out of town.

Patient-centered and family-centered care is far more than just education. It also has to do with how we treat patients. Are we having all of our day-surgery patients and their families show up at 6 a.m. even when we know some of these patients will not have surgery until late morning or early afternoon? If a single mother became ill in the evening, could she schedule a visit with her physician online for the next day so that she could still get her children off to school and know that she could get home in time to be there when the children returned home from school?

Are we engaging patients and their caregivers in the patient's care or still treating the patient as a recipient of care? More than that, are we changing our care processes to activate patients (those with the capacity and competency required) so that they take accountability for their care and use us as consultants and advisors to them?

Nurses and nurse leaders can and must lead this change in the care model together with physicians and other providers.

There will be many new roles for nurses, and the CNO/nurse executive must help develop these roles, help nurses be trained and further educated for these roles, and must develop new ways of assuring the competency of staff for these new nursing roles. Besides the increased use of advanced practice nurses in the team-based care of patients, nurses will have a new and expanded role in population health. We must find ways to promote health and intervene in the lifestyle management and preventive care of those high-risk individuals who are not yet patients. With a movement toward providers assuming greater risk for the health care of a population, the focus will be on trying to avoid costly illnesses and trying to care for those with chronic diseases in the lowest cost environment for which the desired outcomes of care can still be achieved. This means an expansion of home health and palliative care and the development of new roles for nurse educators, patient navigators, and health coaches. Nurses will be even more involved in wellness, prevention, and screenings with special focus on at-risk populations.

Although some primary care and specialist physicians will continue to manage patients with chronic disease in their offices, I believe we will see more chronic disease management being conducted by nurses, physician assistants, advance practice nurses, nutritionists, and other providers in patient-centered medical homes or chronic disease centers of excellence coordinated by teams and evaluated by compliance with evidence-based practices, bundles of care process measures, and metrics of disease management outcomes. The CNO/nurse executive will play a critical role in the design and oversight of these programs.

Finally, I believe that there will be pressure to increase the types of services available to patients at home and work, and for those patients who must be seen, to increase accessibility to care through extended hours of offices/clinics. For those patients who cannot be cared for at home or in an office setting, use of urgent care clinics will be promoted over that of emergency rooms for appropriate cases. This coordination will likely involve more nurse triage and call centers. Finally, for those patients who do end up in hospitals, I believe we will have to move toward true 24/7 operations, a significant challenge for our nurse leaders.

SUMMARY

The CNO/nurse executive is critical to the current executive team and culture and will play an even greater role in redesigning our future health care delivery system. I have been fortunate to have a deep appreciation for the importance of and the role of nursing and have been privileged to work with outstanding nursing leaders at my prior hospital and now in my current health system. Given the knowledge, education, training, experience, caring, and commitment of our nurse leaders, I feel we are well prepared to face the tremendous change and challenges that confront us.

Nursing Leadership: Contributions to Safety and Quality

Al Patterson

Commentary
by Joyce J. Fitzpatrick

*A*s *a clinical pharmacist, Patterson has shared
many experiences with nurses; he reflects on the
key dimensions of nursing leadership and describes
the similarities between the professions of pharmacy
and nursing. One of the most cogent statements he
makes is that nurses are "hard-wired" to be concerned
about patient safety and quality, as are pharmacists.
This value, coupled with a basic professional commitment to patient advocacy for each individual patient
cared for by each nurse, provides the foundation that
distinguishes the professional nurse from other health
professionals.*

*Patterson believes that nursing leaders recognize
the societal responsibility inherent in their role, and
the professional responsibility to provide the most
meaningful care to each patient and to structure the
environment to ensure safety and quality. He continues to delineate the clinical practice and professional
commonalities (e.g., shared governance models, a
full embrace of collaborative practice, and a commitment to evidence-based, data-driven systems) between
nurses and pharmacists, particularly related to the
journeys that both of these professional groups have
experienced in the recent past.*

> *Although pharmacy has recently resolved the professional-entry dilemma by requiring the doctorate for entry into professional practice, nursing has a long way to go to address the professional-entry requirement. Even the recent discussion among nurse leaders regarding the professional doctorate as a requirement for advanced practice has not been implemented and has been strongly criticized as not necessary. Academic nurse leaders could learn from a study of pharmacy education.*

Key focus areas: patient advocacy, professional development, shared governance, collaboration

My first intense exposure to nursing leadership was in the early 1970s while I was a pharmacy intern at Cincinnati Children's Hospital Medical Center (CCHMC). The facility in those days was a strange mix of old and new structures physically interconnected with hallways rife with dark stairwells and basement corridors. As an intern I often worked the evening shifts and usually traveled all the less beaten paths to get around. The director of nursing, Ms. Pauline Heymann, lived on site in a furnished apartment. I literally ran into her in a dark stairwell late one night and this chance encounter scared me to death. I remember her clearly as a paragon of formal professional etiquette. I would frequently cross paths with her as she made her evening rounds dressed in her starched white uniform, a starched white cap, and a blue cape with crimson satin lining. She seemed to be everywhere at all times. My image of her as a nurse leader was somewhat terrifying; it was as if she was omnipresent.

In the winter of 1972, there were a series of patients admitted with unexplained encephalitis, hypoglycemia, and liver failure. All of these patients were desperately ill and their illness was related to post influenza B exposure to aspirin or Reye's syndrome. Then as now, there was no definitive treatment available, but every manner of therapy was initiated, including exchange transfusions, open craniotomies, and drug-induced comas. All of these complicated therapies required a tremendous nursing skill set. I can clearly remember Ms. Heymann standing at a child's bedside with a blood-filled syringe in her hand actually doing the exchange transfusion. Up to that point in my career, I did not think management ever really *did* anything. My vision of nursing changed radically, and more important, my vision of leadership changed as well. She led by doing and this became the foundation of how I would eventually structure my approach to clinical leadership.

> *Not the cry, but the flight of a wild duck, leads the flock*
> *to fly and follow.*
> — ANCIENT CHINESE PROVERB

In over three decades of practice I have had the opportunity to witness the development of a growing collaboration with my nursing colleagues as both of our professions have evolved. The day-to-day professional life of the bedside nurse and the pharmacist share many common elements: the same patients, the same physician colleagues, and the same medication problems. For nursing, the development of a primary care nursing model, implementation of shared governance, and the evolution of the nurse scientist have been but a few of the sea changes that have occurred. Over the same period, my profession has gone through a metamorphosis of professional identity. For pharmacy, the transition from a product-based to a clinical-based profession has been most profound. Simultaneously, both professions have faced unprecedented changes in the structure of health care, including societal, governmental, and financial, which have been totally transformative.

The nursing–pharmacy relationship is always one that is tinged with true collaboration and brother–sister squabbles. But at the core of this relationship is our shared responsibility for the care and well-being of patients. Nursing and pharmacy share a continuous relationship with the patient–family interface daily and both of us work collaboratively in virtually all aspects of the medication process. On the other hand, or so it seems to me, the physician–nurse and physician–pharmacist interactions are usually an intermittent event. The physician assesses diagnoses, prescribes orders, and then walks away. The nurse and the pharmacist are responsible for getting the job done.

My observations and admiration of nursing have evolved over the years. My earliest impressions, aside from my regard for Ms. Heymann, were tinged by the seemingly endless demands of the bedside nurse for services that we did not do well, such as getting the medications there quickly and explaining why their medications were often missing. The focus of the bedside nurse is always on *the* patient; the focus of the pharmacist was on *every* patient—easy to see where conflicts could arise.

There are several things that stand out to me as examples of the transformational nature of nursing leadership: patient advocacy, professional development, and most important, the focus on quality and safety.

PATIENT ADVOCACY

As I matured professionally, I began to recognize that the nurses, all nurses in fact, are motivated by patient advocacy. The nurses were going to do anything and everything necessary to position the patient toward the best outcome. On the other hand, pharmacists had responsibilities that are usually of a greater span by sheer numbers—such that the prioritization of the individual patient was often subservient to the overall prioritization of the many patients in the hospital. Unfortunately, the manner in which the pharmacists dealt with this often engendered a degree of prioritization conflict between nursing and pharmacy. We needed to spend some time in each other's shoes to really understand the difference in our professional priorities.

However, as both professions evolved, recognition that the medication process was an intrinsically shared responsibility between nursing and pharmacy took a while to fully manifest. The nursing staff often took the first step in defining the interprofessional relationship and was usually the first to extend the olive branch of understanding. On the other hand, as pharmacy evolved into a clinical discipline and as pharmacists escaped the basement, the day-to-day interactions between the two professions became genuinely positive and always patient focused.

In the late 1970s, we had a 30-year-old accountant who was involved in a motorcycle accident and fractured his left leg. He developed severe osteomyelitis, requiring around-the-clock intravenous (IV) antibiotic therapy for the normal 6 to 8 weeks.

The patient was otherwise stable and only hospitalized to receive antibiotics. It was now late March, so he was in the middle of tax-preparation season and reportedly, the patient told his surgeon that he would rather have his leg amputated and be allowed to go home rather than to stay in the hospital for the extended IV therapy. This, of course, was in the days before the availability of commercial home IV therapy companies.

The nurse took it upon herself to obtain legal and administrative clearance, as well as commercial insurance coverage. The nurse trained the patient to self-administer the antibiotics and developed a plan for the oversight necessary to safely manage the care of this patient at home. She trained him and documented his competency while arranging for us to provide the medication for home use. She went on to oversee his entire course of therapy. His leg healed, and he is my tax accountant to this day. That nurse taught me what patient advocacy really is: Make it happen for your patients no matter what *it* is.

SAFETY AND QUALITY

Deming's concepts of total quality management (TQM) took hold in health care in the early 1990s. I was given the responsibility for the implementation of TQM principles at CCHMC as well as my usual job—director of pharmacy. The TQM adventure was seen by some as a management fad. The medical staff thought of it as just another flash in the pan or an administration gimmick to control practice variation. In some ways they were right; however, I believe the long-term effect was to establish the primacy of using data in all aspects of day-to-day patient care. The concepts of normal variation, systems thinking, and root cause analysis have stuck with health care since the days of TQM.

TQM focused on the use of quality advisors (QAs) to lead small groups of staff to identify a problem, find the root cause, and establish a structured approach to addressing the problem: the plan–do–check–act mantra. The QAs were trained in small-group dynamics, facilitation, and statistical process control for health care. Initially many department leaders volunteered staff for QA training, and over 160 teams were formed to address a wide array of problems. Over the next 18 months, institutional interest in TQM waned as seems to be a universal phenomenon. For one reason or other, QAs seemed to drop off and were unavailable for assignments, and the remaining QAs were all nurses.

Many of the TQM projects that we took on initially involved a simple process issue such as "why we ran out of paper towels," or "how we can improve missing medication availability," and other important but seemingly short-term issues. Over time the focus of the long-term projects was on improving safety and care delivery. One of the most important gains focused on sepsis associated with the use of central lines. We initially had significant medical participation in the process, but that slowly drifted away and the residual team was entirely composed of nurses and pharmacists. This group identified many of the root causes of central line-associated bloodstream infections and implemented long-term changes that reduced the rate by about 50% from baseline. Mind you, this was in 1993—long before there was universal recognition of the association between central lines and infection. This was a burning example for me that displayed the leadership that nursing has taken in adopting and leading proven scientific methods to improve the quality and safety of care delivery.

I am proud to say that several of the remaining RN QAs have assumed quality leadership positions throughout many large and prestigious academic medical centers. I think it is hardwired into the nurse's soul that quality and patient safety are a core professional responsibility. I think pharmacists share that same DNA thread: we are in this together. In my later career at Children's Hospital Boston, I have had the opportunity to extend my collaboration with nursing leadership as we began the planning and implementation of the electronic clinical information system. The priority for our implementation of the electronic medical record focused on computerized prescriber order entry (CPOE). Early work by David Bates at The Brigham and Women's Hospital promised a significant reduction in medication error rates if CPOE was implemented.

The 1999 Institute of Medicine report, *To Err is Human: Building a Safer Health System* launched the nationwide drive for CPOE implementation and other electronic systems. Our institution had been evaluating potential CPOE vendors for several years prior to *To Err is Human*, but none of the products were developed enough to provide the safety factors necessary for pediatric care. A multidisciplinary leadership team developed a request for a proposal that included CPOE but also included a full closed loop medication management system, including decision-support capability at all steps in the medication management process: prescribing, dispensing, administration, and monitoring. By 2003 we had selected our vendor and began the implementation process. In our justification to the board of trustees for the enormous amount of money that we were requesting for the clinical information system, the return on investment was only based upon reduction in harm associated with adverse drug events (ADEs).

The implementation sequence started with upgrades to the pharmacy and laboratory systems prior to implementation of CPOE. Interestingly, but predictably, our ADE rates did not drop appreciably after these early phases. There was much wringing of hands. From my view, CPOE only eliminated bad handwriting while it did provide some decision-support capability to the prescriber. However, what many had failed to recognize was that in the paper world we still had both the nurse and the pharmacist downstream intercepting the vast majority of prescriber-generated errors.

Clinical information system vendors concentrated much of their development and certainly most of their marketing efforts on meeting the needs of the physician prescriber in the adult setting. Very little effort was directed at providing support for the nurse at the bedside—the last chance to intercept an error before it reaches the patient. Our nursing leadership advocated forcibly and frequently for the development of decision-support capabilities across the entire medication management spectrum.

The final phase of our implementation included full implementation of bedside medication scanning. My nursing leadership colleagues collaboratively took ownership of this phase. A phased implementation with just-in-time data for clinical and leadership staff facilitated adoption of a cultural change regarding barcode scanning. In 12 months our entire institution was converted. Beginning at 6 months into this implementation, the adverse medication event curve began to bend in a positive manner. The curve had remained largely flat after implementation of CPOE. Since the introduction of the bedside scanning, preventable ADEs decreased 50%, and this change has been sustained at the same level for over a year. I attribute a lot of this reduction to the leadership displayed by our nursing colleagues to first advocate for the needed technological application changes and then produce a sustainable cultural change that made it uncool not to scan.

PROFESSIONAL DEVELOPMENT

In 1994 I watched the implementation of a radically different approach to leadership led by my nursing colleagues. Dr. Timothy Porter-O'Grady presented a course-changing lecture on leadership in a clinical setting to the CCHMC staff. The concept of staff empowerment and shared governance rang so true. For the next 18 months, I witnessed the entire course change by my nursing colleagues that led to profound changes at the bedside and, more important, in the careers of the many nursing staff who have been impacted to this day.

The recognition by nursing leadership of the inherent need to provide meaningful control of the care you provide, the environment in which you practice, and your professional development based upon the development and recognition of the societal responsibility of the profession led to all the changes. Pharmacy was undergoing a parallel epiphany as we struggled to define ourselves in a new clinical paradigm: pharmaceutical care—taking responsibility for the therapeutic outcomes of our patients. Pharmacy leadership had historically been hierarchically structured following classic command and control tenets. Leaders led and followers followed with virtually no "managing up" tolerated. The concept that the bedside professional could meaningfully add to the day-to-day direction and, more important, the long-term growth of the profession was a radically new concept.

I am not sure whether the sea change in the nursing leadership (and pharmacy) approach was generated based upon the need to improve recruitment and retention or as a function of the altruistic desire to improve the professional life of staff. Regardless of the cause, the effect was clear: both professions and the patient care provided made quantum leaps.

Central to the concepts of shared leadership/shared governance is the recognition that the profession must continually improve itself. A big elemental part of the improvement was the evolution from diploma-based schools to baccalaureate-trained nurses. Furthermore, at least in my experience in Boston, Cincinnati, and Omaha, it was recognized that nursing leadership needed graduate-level training for advancement into leadership positions. This transformation occurred at an extraordinarily rapid rate, and in less than one decade, a master's degree was widely recognized as a prerequisite to enter formal leadership positions.

At the same time pharmacy was going through a similar conversion; undergraduate pharmacy programs were historically 5-year baccalaureate programs, at least since the mid-1950s. In the 1970s, graduate-level doctor of pharmacy programs focused on the emerging field of clinical practice and were developed primarily on the West Coast and in the Midwest. By the mid-1980s, pharmacy as a profession recognized the need for advanced training for the entry-level professional. In response, the American Council of Pharmaceutical Education adopted the requirement that accreditation would only be awarded to doctoral programs beginning in 1990 and accreditation of bachelor programs would no longer be granted. So the parallels continue between our professions—shared governance and advanced training became the norm for both professions.

It is most impressive to me that the combination of a deep commitment to patient advocacy, a full embrace of collaborative practice models, utilization of a shared governance practice philosophy, and a commitment to evidence-based, data-driven systems has allowed the nursing profession to flourish. My profession has borrowed many leadership cues from our closest colleagues. I personally have stolen many bits of leadership acumen from my nursing sisters; I am a better leader for it.

REFERENCE

Institute of Medicine. (1999). *To err is human: Building a safer health system.* Washington, DC: National Academy Press.

18

"Nursing" Is Not Just About Nurses . . . Nor Is "Leadership" Just About Leaders

Scott Reistad

Commentary
by Joyce J. Fitzpatrick

*R*eistad is a storyteller, and throughout his entry he
entertains readers with his unconventional ideas
about nursing and about leadership. He argues that by
using a definition of nursing that is focused on caring
for the sick and/or infirm, there are many health care
workers who "nurse" others. Those of us in the profession of nursing, perhaps particularly those of us who
are academics, would argue that the definition of nursing needs to be both broader and more precise than that
which Reistad uses. For nursing as professional work
is more than caring. We would agree that to define
nursing as caring requires us to conclude that nursing
is provided by many others, and perhaps by all humans
in some environments and life situations. But this
academic argument misses the most basic and important point that Reistad is making, that is, the extreme
value of person-centered care and meaningful relationships within the care that is provided in health care. All
service providers in health care have a responsibility to
participate in caring in this broader sense.

The second lesson provided by Reistad is
that leadership is about loving the people you lead.
Although this is not a typical definition of leadership,
Reistad describes the results of this leadership style
and encourages aspiring leaders to try it out. He also

> recommends 15 minutes of leadership reading every
> day as a method to learn leadership skills and gain
> understanding. And, importantly, he suggests that
> aspiring leaders associate with those leaders they want
> to emulate, whether or not they are leaders in one's
> own field. Leadership skills carry across professions
> and disciplines, and we are encouraged to learn from
> those who have already demonstrated success.

Key focus areas: love your people, responsive, serve, influence, mentor, world-class

Definition of "nursing":

"A person formally educated and trained in the care of the sick or infirm."

"To look after carefully so as to promote growth, development."

In today's health care, there is a tendency to consider "nursing" as the work of a person who is a registered nurse (RN). Yet as one explores the definitions of "nursing" it becomes obvious that to provide "nursing" is more expansive than this narrowed definition. Who is providing the care to the patient? It would seem that part of investigating this question actually depends on what is considered "care."

- The RN delivers pain medication to the patient who is in pain.
- The respiratory therapist delivers a bronchodilator to the asthmatic patient who is struggling to breathe.
- The laboratory technician draws blood cultures to help determine whether the patient has an infection.
- The nuclear medicine technologist performs a heart scan to determine the condition of the cardiac muscle.
- The physical therapist manipulates the knee of a patient who has recently had surgery.

One can easily see that all of these actions fit the definition of "nursing" as they are each providing patient care.

Now let us expand our horizons a bit.

- The chaplain prays with a patient who is distraught over the diagnosis of cancer.
- The recreational therapist plans activities for the patients who are in the psychiatric unit.
- The financial counselor partners with a family to establish a payment plan for care for their chronically ill child so that they do not have to declare bankruptcy and lose their home.

Not too much of a stretch . . . right?

How about this then:

- The housekeeper, while cleaning the patient's room, begins to talk with a lonely patient.
- The cashier in the cafeteria pays for a family member's meal, when he or she has forgotten to bring money in all of the chaos associated with a loved one coming into the emergency room (ER) as a trauma patient.
- An associate from financial services helps get a distraught, lost family member to the surgery waiting room.
- The volunteer plays cribbage with an elderly Alzheimer's patient.

Aren't these also examples of "nursing"? Aren't these also "looking after and caring for another"?

It seems as if we have relegated "nursing" to the work of the RN when, in fact, caring for patients and their families is a multifaceted process that includes many of the job descriptions within health care. It has been said that all employees in hospitals are caring for patients, either directly or indirectly. There are the individuals who deliver direct patient care . . . and . . . those who support those who give the direct patient care. This delineation seems to much more accurately capture how the "nursing" of a patient takes place.

Many times, one has a tendency to ignore those who support the ones who give the direct patient care until those individuals do not do their jobs. I have found it interesting that one of the primary reasons that hospitals go on ER divert is not that there are not enough RNs . . . or that there is a backup within the computed tomography (CT) department . . . or there is a shortage of medications. A primary cause of divert in many organizations is that of turnaround of a dirty patient room by environmental services. In other words, the entire health care delivery system is hinging on our entry-level wage earner! Does this person even realize how important he or she is?

I remember being invited to a meeting with the transporters of an organization. These individuals moved patients around the organization via wheelchair and gurney . . . had minimal orientation and training and were being paid at the entry-level pay grade. I was to share with their team about the basics of oxygen tank safety and oxygen delivery as many of their patients were using this during their transport. As I shared this information with them, I happened to make this statement: "Your team is one of the most important in the organization." There was a confused look on the faces of many present. One of the transporters raised his hand and said, "I don't understand what you mean. . . . We are only transporters . . . we're not really doing anything important."

I responded by sharing that they are vitally important to the care of these patients. You alone help get patients to tests that can save their lives. You are responsible for their safety. You are there for them when they are filled with anxiety and fear and your talking with them can calm their fears. It was only after I said these things that I began to see a sense of realization for the first time by the transporters that they thought their job was important. Betsy Sanders, a former Nordstrom executive, states that often the lowest paid, shortest-tenured, entry-level employees have more interaction with the patients than the leaders.

When I was a child I had severe asthma symptoms. From about age 5 to 15, I spent about 3 to 4 weeks annually in the hospital. Even as a child, I could distinguish which health care workers truly cared about me and which ones were only "doing their job."

I remember the physician in the ER who shot me with a rubber band and made me laugh when I came in severely wheezing. I recall the transporter who made a game out of "racing" in the wheelchair when I was to go and get an X-ray. I waited for certain nurse assistants who would play games with me. I was judging the care being given to me . . . even as a child . . . by the relationship that these individuals had with me. This impact was so powerful that I actually chose the field of respiratory care as a profession because of a respiratory therapist who inspired me to make a difference.

I frequently use a story to describe how patients are judging the care they receive in the hospital. I have entitled this story the"Car Shop Analogy." How many people, when they go to spend hundreds, if not thousands of dollars, to have their car repaired ask upon arrival, "I'd like to see the continuing education records of the person who is going to work on my car?" No one! Yet who's to say that the person assigned to your car has ever worked on a car like yours? Or experienced a malfunction like the one you are describing? Or maybe is the "worst mechanic in the garage"? Or is a brand-new employee who just finished school and has yet to work on a car? We simply accept that the person who is working on our car is competent and knows what should be done. Why? Interestingly, it is because they are simply employed at the car shop.

Here are my criteria for choosing a car shop:

1. Do they have donuts?

   Reason: I like donuts. And if I am going to have to wait while they repair my car, I'd rather eat donuts than not eat donuts.

2. Will they give me a ride back to my home/work after I drop off my car if the repairs are going to take all day?

   Reason: If I am willing to spend hundreds/thousands of dollars on having my car repaired, they can afford to give me a ride. It annoys me greatly if I have to have my wife tag along behind me in another vehicle to pick me up after I drop my vehicle off . . . and then, to add "insult to injury," I get called and again have to have my wife drive me back down to pick up my car.

3. When they call me to tell me what is wrong with my car, do they use "normal" language so I can understand what is wrong?

   Reason: I really have no idea about how a car works mechanically. In other words, when they say that my "left-handed, counterclockwise turning antigyrational catalytic transmission analyzer" is broken, that is all just gibberish to me. Yet if they would state that "the thing that makes the wheels go round and round is broken"; I would know what that is.

Isn't it interesting that you are probably laughing at my three criteria for choosing a car shop; yet at the same time, I would bet that your criteria . . . though maybe not exactly like mine, probably has similar quirkiness to it? Now think of the patients and how they are choosing which physician, clinic, and hospital is best. The patients and families are judging the care that they are receiving by these criteria:

1. Is the room clean?
2. Is the food warm and tasty?
3. Is my call light answered promptly?
4. Did the doctor smile and talk with me long enough so I could get my questions answered?
5. Am I being treated like a person?

Interestingly, notice how the questions are somewhat similar to those of my criteria for picking a car shop? We think that patients are researching our infection rates, our Joint Commission scores, and the number of complaints that the physicians who take care of them have. Yet, similar to me not asking to see the continuing education records of the car repairman, patients do not ask, "Before you put that IV in, can you show me your competency certificate?" Nor do they ask, "What was your score on your national exam?" Leapfrog with me to some of the questions that are being asked of patients by the Hospital Consumer Assessment of Health Providers and Systems, as part of value-based purchasing:

1. How often did nurses treat you with courtesy and respect?
2. How often did nurses explain things in a way you could understand?
3. During this hospital stay, after you pressed the call button, how often did you get help as soon as you wanted it?
4. How often was the area around your room quiet at night?

Aren't these reminiscent of how I chose my car shop?

"Nursing" is encompassing so many other aspects of care besides just the technical part of the job . . . and is also including many other people besides those with the credential of "RN."

So what are patients looking for in their "nursing" care? I would suggest that they are looking for what I entitle a "*wow!*" experience.

What is "*wow!*"? "*Wow!*" has a definition of a person being amazed . . . astonished . . . overwhelmed. Of someone stating, "I can't believe that they would have done that for me!"

"*Wow!*" is different for each individual patient and family member. What *wow!*s one patient may not *wow!* another.

I am betting that you can think of *wow!* experiences in your life when a restaurant, hotel, business, school, church, or someone did something for you that was not just good . . . not just great . . . but *wow*!

Let me recount a story for you that may illustrate what I am talking about. I know that many of you have been to Disneyland and have experienced the magic of the place. Before going, I had read many Disney books and articles and knew of their reputation of delivering extraordinary care and service to their guests. Yet to know it and to experience it are two different things.

A friend had recommended to me to make sure that I had an "Apple Pie Apple" while at Disneyland. For those who are unaware of what this delicacy is all about, let me describe its deliciousness to you: It is an apple that is first dipped in caramel . . . then re-dipped in white chocolate . . . then rolled in cinnamon and sugar . . . and finally doused in pie-crust crumbs. Yum!

Well, we had been enjoying Disneyland, when I suddenly remembered that I was to purchase one of these delectable items. Now, not knowing where I could purchase one of these, I had remembered that the cast members (as their employees are called at Disney) who are responsible for the trash clean-up are given extensive orientation to know where everything is located. So, in looking around, I spied one of them nearby.

I walked over and asked, "Excuse me, but could you point me toward where I could get an 'Apple Pie Apple'"?

His response was a bit atypical, but in retrospect, perfectly Disney-esque.

He stated, "Oh my gosh! Those are awesome!"

He then said to me, "Alright everyone . . . follow me!"

I stated, "No, I see you are busy, just kind of point me in the direction I am to go and I can find it on my own."

He would have nothing to do with this. Instead, he swooped up me and my family and off we went toward what he told me was Pooh Corner (which for those of you who are familiar is behind the Log Ride in Frontier Land!)

This cast member began chatting with me and my family.

"Where are you from?"

"How long are you here?"

"What have you liked best so far?"

"Have you done this yet?"

"I'd highly recommend this activity/place/attraction."

Before we knew it, we had traversed the park and were at Pooh Corner. Before departing, he thanked us. . . . Yes . . . thanked us for allowing him to serve us and make recommendations.

Therefore, an "ordinary" experience becomes a *wow!* experience because of the caring and service demonstrated by this person.

I am sure that you can recall a time when a restaurant/hotel/ store/service did something that made you say *wow!* It may have been bending over backward to accommodate a special request. It might have been demonstrating to you that you are "special." It might have even been an amazing service recovery when things did not go the way that they were originally supposed to. In fact, as you recall this event(s), these are often the stories that you like, and even want, to share with others. The stories that begin with, "Hey, you won't believe this when I tell you, but company ABC did this for me when. . ."

As you recall these inspiring actions, think back as to how the *wow!* came into being. No doubt it was the actions of a single person. It was someone who made the choice to "go the extra mile" for you. And yet, we most often think of the event as being done by the company and not the individual employed by the company. The power we have as an individual to demonstrate extraordinary caring and service is within each one of us. We . . . not the company . . . are what make the *wow!* happen. Conversely, it only takes the actions of one associate to also demonstrate "non *wow!*" behavior too.

Our patients and families are most likely not expecting much from their health care experience. Over the years, they have been so regularly disappointed in our care and service as we have treated them as a diagnosis or as a room number.

"Can you go and check the fresh appendectomy for me . . . their light is on again."

"427 wants to go to the bathroom."

As we transition to caring for the patient as a person . . . Robert . . . Jennifer . . . Mr. Adams . . . Mrs. Williams . . . and begin to see them as a rock climber, a father, a school teacher, a daughter . . . as a person who is frightened . . . angry . . . sad . . . it is then, and really only then, that we have the ability to extend *wow!* to them.

John Murphy states that "Customers no longer compare you to your direct competition. Customers now compare you to every supplier and service provider they come in contact with. The rules have changed. If a customer has been 'wowed' by someone else, they wonder why they cannot experience the same thing with you. Consciously or subconsciously, fairly or unfairly, people compare you to every other business they buy from. Stop for a moment and ask yourself, is your business FedEx-fast and Disney-friendly? Is your team Nordstrom-aware and Amazon-efficient?"

As the American health care culture continues to change, those health care organizations that are unable to provide these *wow!* experiences, as other companies do, will quite abruptly discover that they have been left behind and are out of business.

As we transition to discuss the issue of leadership, the most challenging fact is that of this axiom: "World-class employees *only* want to be a part of a department/organization with world-class leaders."

Who is a leader? What is leadership?

I think John Maxwell states it best in two of his famous quotes:

"Leadership is influence."
"He who thinks he leads, but has no followers, is only out taking a walk."

Many still believe that leadership is a title . . . but think about someone you know who has a "title" and yet has little influence and few, if any, followers. Continue the exercise by thinking of others who do not have a "title" and yet seem to have great influence and followers. Leadership comes in many shapes and forms.

What health care, like many other industries, seems to struggle with is realizing that extraordinary technical skills do not equate to extraordinary leadership skills. Sure, there can be a correlation as it can be challenging for an RN to follow a leader who has no medical background. But if one fulfills the expectations of having influence and having followers, why is a degree or title a limitation?

I recall from my employment at a hospital where the "unthinkable" occurred. There came an opening for the manager of the anesthesia department. Upon analysis of the skill set that was needed to help move the anesthesia department to the next level, it was determined that at this juncture they needed a person with a great deal of logistical, organizational, quality, and process expertise. So my boss chose an individual who had an MBA (master of business administration) instead of a person from the anesthesia department . . . or even with a medical background!

One would have thought that the world was coming to an end when the decision was announced.

"How can she lead us? She doesn't know anything about what we do!"

"She's just a 'bean-counter'!"

"What is administration thinking? Are they really that stupid?"

Yet this person came in, honestly shared that she was unfamiliar with much of the terminology and what employees did. She went about her job humbly and respectfully. She listened and learned. She asked lots of questions.

She identified issues for which she could partner with others to help resolve. She asked for help. She was responsive. She delegated issues that she believed others could do better. Over time, she became an extraordinary leader with a great deal of influence from physicians, CRNAs, OR (operating room) techs, and others. Thus, she proved that leadership need not have technical expertise so long as there are those who do have that expertise.

As the term "leader" is used, the natural tendency is to think of titles: director, manager, supervisor, lead, charge, and so on. Yet according to the definition of "having influence" and "having followers," this easily refers to many other individuals in the organization.

I am sure you are aware of the term "informal leader," but that does not mean that the person has any less power and authority than a person who has a title and is considered a "formal leader."

I joined an organization in which there were some extraordinarily strong leaders who did not have titles. When I was more naïve about leadership and felt that I had to control everything, the first thing that I did was to assert my positional authority.

"Hey! Listen to me! I'm the Director!"

Which . . . as you would guess . . . got me exactly nowhere.

Through mentoring, I was instructed to instead use the informal leader's power as a way of extending my leadership power. By asking questions of these leaders, I discovered amazing insights that they had. I found that they had power because they deeply care about what is going on in the department. I found out that at times I had good ideas . . . but at other times, I was just flat-out wrong.

I discovered that there was some truth to the old saying, "If you can't beat them, join them." Yet in fact, I was not really trying to "beat them" at all. Instead, we learned to partner with one another.

This was very challenging for me . . . and at times . . . still is.

As I look at promoting one of my team members to be a "formal" leader, I advocate that they must already possess leadership skills *before* they are promoted. The best leaders are not leaders who become so when they put on their new name tag. Instead, they are the people who are already seen as leaders by their peers even when they do not have a formal title.

Years ago, I was developing a new subspecialty area in the respiratory care department I was overseeing. I needed to have a coordinator in the area, so I developed a job description and posted the position. I had a number of applicants, including the therapist who had the strongest clinical skills in the area, apply.

At the interview, I asked all of the candidates this question: "Describe to me how you are demonstrating leadership skills right now that are making an impact in the area." The therapist who had the strongest clinical skills answered this way: "I have no leadership skills right now. But you realize that I know the most in the area, so if you simply promote me, I'll really start to show you what kind of leader I am." As you would guess, he had already demonstrated his leadership skills by his lack of being a leader where he was already working.

So that brings us to those of us who have "titles." We have a huge responsibility to be/become amazing leaders! I regularly share with others that once they have accepted the mantle of leadership, they take on the expectation of life long learning. For unlike doing a technical job, where there may be a "perfect" way to do a task (Take A and twist it onto B . . . then insert it into C), dealing with people is unique in every interaction.

"Nursing" leaders have a tendency to have read thousands of pages of textbooks about the technical aspects of their job. Yet they get promoted into leadership and believe that they should just magically know what to do to lead effectively. I am guessing that you may have heard this quote:

Question: "What happens when you promote an extraordinary bedside nurse to be a leader?"
Answer: "You get a terrible manager and lose a good nurse."

"Nursing" leaders need to commit to growing themselves to become *wow!* leaders so that they have the opportunity to attract, retain, and lead *wow!* associates.

I am betting that you may have seen or experienced this scenario: An amazingly talented employee is successfully recruited into the organization to work on a specific unit. The person arrives filled with expectations that were shared with them by Human Resources and the department manager. As the person works more days on the unit, she begins to see that the manager is "over her or his head" in being able to lead effectively. The manager has little trust in the department. The manager is disorganized. The manager has favorites. The manager does not follow up on questions or concerns. The employee begins to become more and more disgruntled . . . and finally, either becomes disaffected and disengaged or chooses to leave the organization.

How are leadership skills grown? I have found that it is really through two key components: reading and association. Reading and association help a person to enhance her or his leadership skills more quickly and easily by not having to learn everything on his or her own and to not have to make all of the errors.

Let us start by talking about books.

With the myriad of leadership books that are in print (simply go to the management/leadership section of your local bookstore and you will see what I mean!), what books should I read? My suggestion is to first ask your supervisor if she or he has recommendations. Quite possibly the supervisor may have some books that have influenced the supervisor greatly, which will be a great place for you to get started.

In choosing a leadership book to read, I think that one of the most important aspects is that it must be interesting to you! If you are struggling to read the book, maybe this is a book for later. Set it aside and get something else. If you are reading something that is fun, the time spent reading flies by.

I realize that I am somewhat "atypical" in that I love to read, whereas many made a vow not to read anything besides the newspaper, magazines, and Facebook after finishing school. Here is an easy suggestion to help you develop the reading habit: "Nursing" leaders need to read at least 15 minutes per day . . . every day.

I can hear it already:

"I'm so busy I don't have time to read"
"I don't like to read."
"I have kids and they never leave me alone long enough to read."

Unfortunately, excuses are not part of the equation, so let me again state the expectation: "Nursing" leaders need to read at least 15 minutes per day . . . every day.

Here is a tip that can help. There is a private place that everyone goes to every day . . . sometimes even twice . . . where you sit down . . . all alone . . . in a locked room . . . where you would be able to get 15 minutes of time to read if you put your book there.

I have become somewhat of a leadership mentor to many with whom I work and a frequent question I get asked is "How do you know all of this stuff?" When I tell them that I read 15 minutes per day they look unimpressed. Then I tell them that I have been doing so for 31 years. I have read hundreds of books on leadership, human behavior, marriage relationships, positive mental attitude thinking, goal setting, conflict management, and so on. I am not a leadership savant . . . I have simply plodded along for many years learning a little bit at a time. You can, too, by simply beginning to grow your leadership skills through reading.

My next suggestion is to associate with other leaders/mentors.

My leadership mentor made this statement, which has always stuck with me: "You can either learn from folks who have already made the mistakes and are trying to help you avoid the same mistakes . . . or . . . you get to make all the mistakes on your own and learn from them. It's a lot easier and faster to not have to repeat all of the errors . . . but it is your choice."

The caveat is this: Associate with those leaders you wish to emulate. I realize that you might think that you should hang around with other health care leaders because they are in your same unit . . . have a similar title as you (Clinical Nurse Manager, for example). But the same advice you give your kids is true as an adult too: "Those you hang around with are those whom you will become like." If you hang around with "mediocre" leaders, you will learn "mediocre" leadership skills. But conversely, if you hang around extraordinary, amazing leaders, you will then pick up these traits as well.

Do not even limit yourself to those leaders who are in your same field. The leadership skills of others in the other service industries can inspire you to greatness in "nursing" leadership. What could you learn if you took a leader from the Imaging department out to lunch? Environmental Services? What about a supervisor you know from Barnes and Noble? Or Red Lobster? How about your pastor? The president of your Home Owners Association?

Leadership skills have many commonalities across all industries. The responsibility of leadership is to be a servant to those whom you lead. "Nursing" leadership is no different.

Lastly, your staff will buy into you as their leader well before they buy into the vision that you are attempting to articulate. As mentioned previously, leaders have followers. Followers do so voluntarily. You must work to make yourself "attractive" to your people. This is not to manipulate them, but instead to serve them better.

A few years ago, I had an MBA student who was being assigned to various leaders around the organization as part of her practicum. She ended up with me during a very challenging time during which I ended up being an "interim" leader for another department far outside my "comfort zone" of Respiratory Care.

We had been working to lead this department for a number of weeks when one day she said to me, "I've been with a number of leaders during my time here at the hospital, and I can't seem to really figure you out."

I was puzzled by this statement and asked her what she meant.

She stated, "Well, I've been in a number of departments around the organization, and you do things so differently than many other leaders. You get things done in a different way. . . . People seem to respond to you differently. . . . People are willing to do things that I would normally think that they would balk at . . . and people seem to work harder than I'd think they would. I've been watching and I can't seem to figure out what you are doing that's making them act like this."

It was then that I shared with this soon-to-be health care leader the "secret formula" to leading people. I told her, "You must truly, truly love your people. Not as a way of manipulating them to get them to do things your way. Not as a gimmick. Not through some techniques that you have learned in your schooling. But to really, really love them as persons. This is the essence of leadership. People can tell if you are 'faking it.' But they can also tell if you truly are living it out. The greatest leaders always love their people and that is why they are able to have so much influence and have so many followers."

There was a quizzical look. Then a very long pause. Then she just walked away as what I had said did not align with all of the techniques and the papers and the lectures that she had attended while striving for her MBA.

I had failed.

Months later she left my oversight and graduated. She got a job in health care leadership. I have heard that she is frustrated by her job as it has so many people problems. Instead, she wants to move to a job that is much more about "projects" . . . in other words, not people.

The quintessential point of "nursing" leadership . . . in fact; any kind of leadership . . . is this: Love your people.

By loving your people, they will grow beyond your expectations and soar to heights that you never could have imagined. They will lift your department. They will bring accolades to your organization. They will *wow*! your patients and families.

Through it all, they may bring you tears of joy . . . and tears of heartbreak.

Relationships with people is what life is about. Why must one separate caring for others to those only outside of work?

Yes, I know that this is not what is always taught in school or even by other leaders.

There are those who appear to be "successful" and seem to get the results required, but this is all just temporary if one does not have relationships with and love for those whom one has been gifted to lead.

For you see ... to be an amazing, extraordinary, *wow*! "nursing" leader, you only need to strive to be one of the greatest servers and greatest lovers of people.

19

Nurse Leadership

Anne Rosewarne

Commentary
by Joyce J. Fitzpatrick

*R*osewarne has a wealth of experience working
with nurses at all levels in many different roles.
*During more than two decades as president of the
Michigan Health Council, she has seen many changes
in the demands on nurse leaders and others in the
health care industry. Accordingly, she advises nurse
leaders to embrace the changes.*

*Roswarne is particularly attuned to workforce
issues in nursing, and the Council has developed
specific programs to address the challenges of nurse
turnover. Through the Council a leadership development program was established, focused primarily on
preparing nurse managers as leaders within their
health care facilities. The participants have identified
many areas of growth, including changes in attitudes
and behaviors, knowledge and skill acquisition, self-
awareness, and team-building skills. The program
includes inspirational and motivational components,
which, according to Rosewarne, are important dimensions to developing leaders. Thus, passion for nursing,
leadership, and, more generally, health care delivery,
are renewed, and nurse leaders are supported through
the program leaders and through their peers.*

*There are a number of key changes that are
occurring now that Rosewarne considers important for nurse leaders to understand. These include*

> *changes in health policy and practices, succession planning, diversity issues as the makeup of the population changes, and the new Doctor of Nursing Practice programs. Rosewarne advises nurse leaders to understand policy and finance issues in health care in order to be more effective in their roles.*

Key focus areas: embrace change, team member, partnerships, strategic vision

When asked to write a chapter on the future of leadership in nursing, I readily agreed. I have been president of the Michigan Health Council (MHC) for the past 21 years and in that role as the director of MHC, I have had the opportunity to work with nurses from all facets of nursing, education, practice, and policy. In particular, for the past 10 years my organization has been contracted by the state to manage the Michigan Center for Nursing, so I have observed and learned from many nursing leaders and watched nursing leadership grow and flourish. Our very capable director, Carole Stacy, MSN, MA, RN, has started and implemented many innovative programs designed to promote leadership in nursing. This focus has allowed me to ruminate on the nexus between workforce and nursing, illuminating the importance of nursing leadership to the future of an increasingly complex health care system. The MHC serves as a convener and catalyst for the health care workforce in the state. The Council's many programs range from managing Health Occupations Students of America (HOSA), a high school student organization to promote career opportunities and quality health care, to revenue-generating job boards for health professionals to an Internet-based clinical placement tool with a passport function that coordinates the regulatory requirements for a student entering a clinical placement. Our focus at MHC is to build sustainable programs that address the workforce with new technology, new models of care, and clearer insight into workforce issues in the state. As MHC's primary focus is the health care workforce, these years have been interesting years indeed. We have seen *sweeping* changes to the health care system, and therefore, to the entire workforce, but particularly to the nursing profession.

LEADERSHIP

My own ideas of leadership in general have grown from my past experience working in the nonprofit community. I became an Association leader at a transition time for nonprofits. The days of the top-down, autocratic leader were ushered out partially by the Information Technology industry, with its horizontal organization chart and teamwork focus. Leaders now are being chosen for having very different qualities than in the past. Even so, the main challenge is still negotiating the misalignment of people's needs with organizational needs. Addressing employee's needs and abilities are a crucial component of a successful organization, and leaders are increasingly being evaluated on their ability to stimulate, facilitate, and reward and retain employees. In order to be productive in today's global environment, leaders, including nurse leaders, must embrace this change.

PROMOTING LEADERSHIP IN NURSING

My understanding of leadership in nursing is based on MHC's many efforts to support Michigan's 160,000 nurses through surveys, research, conferences, trainings, educational programs, and support to all Michigan nursing organizations. For example, we at MHC have learned that when nursing leaders learn to more effectively manage and administrate, it can improve the quality of care. Our Michigan Center for Nursing Survey 2008 found that 21% of nurses left their current nursing position in the last 2 years. Almost half (41%) of those responding said a major influence in their decision to leave was a lack of job satisfaction related to a poor relationship with their manager or administration. This amount of turnover places effective, safe patient care at risk, because when nurses leave, a vacuum is created until another nurse fills that position. It may be weeks or months until a nurse is hired and more months until that nurse is oriented to the system and can carry a full patient assignment competently. During the time it takes to fill the vacant position and orient the new hire, the rest of the nursing staff is assuming a larger patient care load, maybe working longer hours and more days, which leads to increased errors and decreased time for each patient. Turnover is also costly for an organization's recruitment and training resources and may waste limited nursing education resources. Given these survey results, we felt Michigan needed a program to provide nursing leaders with the necessary leadership skills to create a stable care environment.

To address this need, we believed the place to begin was with the position of the nurse manager. In January 2010, the Michigan Center for Nursing submitted a Partners Investing in Nursing grant proposal titled *Leading Toward Tomorrow*. The grant was funded by Robert Wood Johnson, Blue Cross/Blue Shield of Michigan, and Community Foundation of Southeast Michigan. The goal of this project was to develop a pipeline of educated, talented clinical leaders to staff Michigan's health care organizations. The role of competent and skilled clinical leaders is not only critical to the delivery of high-quality, safe, and reliable care for patients, but also contributes to the overall performance of their units and the organization. The nurse manager, in particular, is in the unique position to affect care delivery at the patient level wherever and whenever it occurs. The purpose of the *Leading Toward Tomorrow* project was to design, implement, and evaluate a comprehensive Leadership Development Program (LDP) that would assist in a nurse's leadership growth. The program was designed to assist nurses in gaining new and different skills and competencies as well as improving and enhancing current ones to facilitate their leadership development journey.

The curriculum included 8 days of face-to-face sessions spaced over 4 months and was designed to help nurse managers develop the skills needed to provide a stable work and care environment. Specifically, it included in-depth information on health care finance and reimbursement, patient quality and safety, dealing with difficult employees, creating a just and accountable culture, managing change, project planning and business plan development, along with creating a positive work environment, and hiring with the thought of retention. Participants were asked to create a project that would speak to one of these areas and improve the work on their units. They were assigned mentors and coaches to assist with the project.

From this effort, we have learned that these leadership skills empower nurse managers. Thus far, three cohorts of nurse managers participated in the pilot program for a total of 128 participants. Yet to be completed is a 6-month postprogram evaluation for cohort two and cohort three. Individual postprogram evaluations have shown that participants felt more comfortable in their role as managers because of the information they had acquired. The areas they thought were most beneficial were finance, creating a just culture, and dealing with staff attitude problems. In the words of participants, here is how they evaluate the leadership:

- I have been very aware of my own management style, but it was good to get confirmation. It was especially valuable to identify other managers' styles and their effect on my day-to-day operations. It was helpful to identify attitudes and behaviors that undermine my style decreasing the culture in my facility. Also, I felt the speaker's contribution was very valuable regarding accountability and dealing with attitude problems of staff. It was also very interesting to examine generational differences.
- An amazing leadership opportunity. This is the information I have been seeking!
- Self-assessment—identifying my biggest leadership challenges and areas for growth. A great time for reflection—a step back—to have a new perspective on leadership.
- Sparked new ideas on multiple tasks I am going to have to complete on my unit. Helped me to realize that I can do this.
- Knowing that I was not the only person new to a leadership position, and we are all learning together. Creating an open discussion on day one made me more comfortable.
- Being with other leaders, wow, sometimes I feel totally alone but now I see my network forming.
- It was a distinct privilege to be a part of this initial Leading Toward Tomorrow (LTT) consortium. To rub shoulders with exceptional nursing leaders and to hear their perspectives is something I will treasure professionally.
- This is a fabulous program. I have learned so much. Now I feel I have the tools to start on my journey to be an awesome leader. The leaders *were very inspirational*. I will be starting classes for BSN (bachelor of science in nursing) in March and plan on pursuing my master's degree. I would recommend this program to all nurse leaders. I feel very privileged to be a part of this conference. *In listening to so many amazing speakers, I have found a new passion in nursing leadership.* Thank you so much.

We have also learned that nursing leadership can be promoted through personal and motivational experiences. Twice a year for the last six years, 40 nurses from around the state, representing small and large employers, go up to Michigan's beautiful North Country to hear inspirational and challenging speakers and rejuvenate around a crackling bonfire. The nurses talk about what is important to them, their careers, their dedication, job issues, and health care trends at the Michigan Institute of Nursing Excellence. Although billed as a reenergizing experience for bedside nurses, not for building leadership, many nurses have written a year or two later to profess the impact of being with other nurses from all walks of nursing and hearing inspirational speakers sent them home to do many new and challenging things; it changed them into leadership thinkers. Following are some of the nurse comments after attending the Institute:

- The Institute of Nursing Excellence gave me the ability to be vulnerable and very open with others who are strangers, but kindred in a spirit and profession that binds us. I saw a lot of emotion, passion, and excitement.
- Team building and learning to think outside the box are frequently required to complete a shift in my job—thank you for assisting in this.
- This week has really renewed my passion for nursing and been such a rejuvenating time. I *loved* talking to the other nurses about their work and organizations. Energizing, encouraging—life changing. *Thank you so much!!*
- Very inspiring for me to know the nurses of Michigan have a very strong leadership presence at the top! You all have inspired me to one day → be there. ☺ Thank you!
- Enlightening! Empowering! Totally awesome! I can't wait to take this back to my organization. Truly a life-changing experience!
- I have lots of ideas and thoughts to take back to our facility to help improve or promote change. I think this (for me) has been a very positive experience and reinforced my role as RN (registered nurse). It's unique, important, professional, and functional, and I can use it for self, patient, and others.
- An experience I won't soon forget. It's nice to realize we are all concerned about similar things, we all have a passion for nursing, and that I work at a pretty progressive and good place, makes me really appreciate what I have.
- Magnificent. It regained my strengths, confidence, and my goals for the future.

CHALLENGES FOR THE FUTURE OF LEADERSHIP
AND NURSING

I think there has never been a better time for nurse leaders to move forward. The national and state changes in the delivery and reimbursement systems will continue, with nurses poised as well-trained, cost-effective leaders in the shortage-ridden primary care workforce. We will need nurse leaders at every point of entry in the existing health care system and will find their skills and understanding a vital component in building a more patient-centered model in the health care workforce. However, in present-day health care, change and innovation make everything happen faster. There are plenty of opportunities for not only great successes, but also great challenges and even failures.

The Affordable Care Act

In the next 10 years, nurse leaders will be in an enviable position as health care changes roll out from the Affordable Care Act (ACA); I do see some challenges for them, however. The implementation of ACA will do one thing immediately: it will make us acutely aware of the shortages in the entire primary care team. For some time there has been a Paul Revere warning from medical groups that there was a shortage of primary care physicians before ACA that is now exacerbated by the Act. There is a concomitant shortage of advance practice nurses, many of whom are moving to acute care settings. Acute care is appealing to nurse practitioners and doctors of nursing practice (DNPs) because of the regular hours, "no call" policy, autonomy, and a favorable work environment. A 2010 MHC-commissioned study in Michigan demonstrated that 31% of advanced practice nurses now practice in acute care settings, which is a significant increase from 5 years ago. When conversation about primary care shortages comes up, the solution is always to employ nurse practitioners (NPs), DNPs, and physician assistants (PAs) to accommodate the shortfall. However, there is simply not enough of either to quickly fill the gap. Ramping up educational programs is difficult because of already serious faculty shortages, decreasing availability of clinical sites, and shortage of lab and classroom space.

However, nurse leaders from colleges and universities all over the United States have been creatively stepping up to address this impending critical nursing shortage by increasing enrollment and establishing short-term completer degrees for students with an existing undergraduate degree. The nurse leaders are also doing two important things that all leaders must do—share and communicate.

The New Doctor of Nursing Practice

The nursing councils and committees nationwide shared resources and best practices, paving the way for other schools to ramp up enrollment to meet burgeoning health care industry needs. The leaders also communicated both privately and publicly about their efforts. When leaders collaborate and communicate, particularly in a nonprofit environment, everyone wins. Nurse leaders have recently created the doctor of nursing practice as a terminal degree in nursing. The DNP focus is on clinical practice rather than academic research. Nurse leaders recognized the accelerating workforce needs in primary care accompanied by the 21st century demand for health care outpacing the supply of doctors and other health professionals. As the United States and the world have more resources, chronic disease from lifestyle choices plus aging present new challenges that the 20th-century models of care are not suited to deliver efficiently or effectively. Nurses will be asked to delegate, cooperate, and participate on teams of care. Coaching, patient education, and follow-up will emerge as critical components of containing cost and delivering effective results-based health care. Nurse leaders must educate the health care workforce and the public about the DNP so they understand the scope of practice and where the DNP fits into the hierarchy of health professions.

Evidence-Based Practices

Nurses use evidence-based practice (EBP) to make clinical decisions. EBP involves complex and conscientious decision making based not only on the available evidence but also on patient characteristics, situations, and preferences. It recognizes that health care is individualized and ever changing and involves uncertainties and probabilities. As both leaders and hands-on caregivers, nurses have always advocated for EBP with the patient at the center. Increasingly, nurses will be relied on to observe, cultivate, teach, and learn from EBP, with their awesome responsibility of around-the-clock vigilance for patients, their voice is integral to building our improved system. There are new opportunities for nurse educators to promote testing and adopting of new health care policies.

Collaboration

New opportunities in an evolving health care system will also include nurses engaging as team members in interprofessional (IPE) settings. For all health professionals, this presents a real conundrum: Who is the leader of an IPE group? Do we need a leader? How does each professional function as a team yet still retain professional skills and scopes? Does the facilitator need to be a health professional? My main observation about this team phenomenon is that *everyone* wants to be the leader, which does not really work. Some of the best models of IPE exist outside of the United States. The University of Toronto has been a leader in team training both in academics and in practice. Their teams evolve with each participant leading the effort for their profession but no "team leader," per se. A facilitator keeps conversation and communication at a professional, effective level but does not lead the team in relation to patient issues. I think the primary leadership challenge in IPE is for advance practice and RN and BSN nurses to firmly establish nursing in a pivotal position and still be a good team player.

Succession Planning

As the nursing workforce ages, we must do everything we can to retain seasoned nurse leaders as a contributing resource. With age often comes a degree of common sense and a willingness to speak up and we do not want to lose the benefits of all that "ripening." Although everyone agrees succession planning is crucial, it often is not implemented and does not plan for emergencies. There has been some change in both academics and practice to accommodate the aging workforce, but we need more.

Understanding Policy Issues

One of the greatest needs in health care is for nurses who understand policy issues. We need nurses with degrees in business, public policy, or law as well as nursing to reach across the professions and develop partnerships. My observation is that we have very few nurses who are well versed in policy development and implementation. We need more nursing leadership on nursing education funding, practice issues, and IPE practice. More nurse policy leaders could empower nurses and develop a new generation of nurse leaders. Nurse policy leaders could develop in-depth understanding of other members of the health care team, their practice parameters, and relevant health policy issues. Nurse policy leaders could join with other professions to draft legislation that would help not only the patient but all professions. They could help frame reimbursement and quality and safety discussions. They could train all nurses to understand the arduous process of drafting, advocating, and implementing new legislation.

Understanding Health Care Finance

As I think about encouraging more nurses to move into leadership positions, gaining an understanding of health care financing from A to Z is essential. In our future plans in health care, we will all pay special attention to the quality of care and outcomes, and we have embraced that as a necessary component of future health care delivery. What does not receive equal attention and commitment is a thorough understanding of health care finance. Nurses should know how health care is paid for: How much is paid by Medicare? Medicaid? Private Insurance? How much of health care is unpaid, and how does it vary? How will it change with the ACA? Where are these savings or economies of scale that nurses could implement both small and big? Can we save time using new technology, procedures, and ideas? Are there ways to streamline administrative tasks? Are we delegating when appropriate? And most important, are we duplicating efforts repeating information unnecessarily either to a patient or coworker? I do know how cost conscious nurses can be, and I wonder how much more could be applied in a work setting with nurse leadership.

Diversity

While the United States becomes more diverse, the nursing workforce shows some improvement in adding diversity, but not enough to match the population. Nursing schools are challenged to be academically rigorous and apply the same standards of acceptance to all incoming students; therefore students from superior high schools compete for the open slots. Nursing requires both science and math skills, which are often a roadblock for a person returning to the workforce or a student from a less competitive high school. Diverse involvement is also low among nurse leaders both in practice and academia. In Michigan, only 6% of our registered nurse population is African American and 4% are Asian, 1% American Indian, and 2% Latino. This does not reflect our population distribution at all. Programs to address this gap can be effective, but there are not enough of them to create real growth and the programs are often terminated when grant funding ends.

INSPIRING NURSE LEADER

For me, it is perhaps easiest to visualize the future of nursing leadership by thinking of an old friend of mine who not only fully understood the issues I have just described but also embodied the values of nurse leadership. Over the years, I have worked with many inspiring nurse leaders, but Carol Franck, ex-CEO (chief executive officer) of the Michigan Nurses Association (MNA), stands out for me as the ultimate leader. Carol chose the nursing profession because of the intellectual challenge and the opportunity to make a difference in people's lives. She always lent her beacon-intensity intellect to problems and issues and came out with cogent thoughts and a clear direction. Carol strategized and initiated public policy positions and legislation that was adopted or passed. She was instrumental in establishing mandatory continuing medical education for all nurses, diversion for disciplined nurses, the Nurse Professional Fund for scholarships and research, durable power of attorney guidelines, and political action committees (PACs) for nursing policy. Carol understood her role as leader of the MNA clearly. She was able to maintain balance of the many constituent groups in the MNA. When Carol was on duty there was always a clarion call for access to care for vulnerable populations. She was vocal about nursing salary levels, scope of practice limitations, the need for nurses to organize and be paid a competitive wage, and she advocated for adequate funding for nursing education.

Establishing and holding a pivotal position for nursing among the health professions was important to Carol. She always gave all professions respect and looked for common ground and accord with them. She did not engage in pettiness or backbiting and was *always* honest about her position. Carol Franck had a strategic vision and she steered toward it unfailingly. She was creative, a risk taker, inspiring, and a great communicator. I think of her often when there is an unarticulated issue in the room or when tact is not the first response anyone thinks of. She would handle it, and so do some of us who were lucky enough to glean some of her honesty and wisdom. When Carol retired to New York and Cape Cod, I gave her Annie Leibovitz's (1999) book *Women* and noted that she deserved a page in there all of her own. I thought she easily matched Leibovitz's subjects in brains and accomplishments. Several years later, Carol died, leaving all of us with memories and deeply ingrained lessons of tact and how to exhibit patience, along with willingness for a good fight if conditions arose.

So whether it is looking to the past for an inspirational leader or attaching substantive issues like practice models, diversity cost, EBP, delegation, or IPE practice and education, nurses are uniquely positioned to be an integral part of the change and to lead us to a health care system that is both efficient and cost-effective.

REFERENCE

Leibovitz, A., & Sontag, S. (1999). *Women*. New York, NY: Random House.

Nursing, Health Reform, and the Achievement of Better Health for All People

Barry H. Smith

Commentary
by Joyce J. Fitzpatrick

*S*mith's opening is significant: that nursing care is at the core of humanity. He recounts his own experiences with nurses, when as a surgical resident he learned the value of team work, and developed a respect for the nurses who were so tuned in to the needs of the patients and families. He also points to this experience as the place in which he learned both the true nature of nursing and the unrealized potential of nursing.

Smith asserts that nurses must be the central point of any health care system, and yet many factors have converged to keep nurses in a subservient role within health care. Yet, he asserts that nurses must be the interface between people and health, as both caregivers and facilitators. To enact their central role nurses must be societal leaders and activists. This is a key lesson to be communicated to nurse leaders at all levels. Societal activists are involved, seen, and heard. They are at the table, speaking, and leading. They are not comfortable with the status quo, but are pushing health care forward on behalf of people everywhere. They are involved in their communities.

Smith delineates the many roles that nurses as leaders in health care can assume. He argues for the centrality of nursing in the redesign of the U.S. health

> *care system. He describes nurses as the beating heart of a health care system, serving the people and ensuring quality of life for all.*

Key focus area: unleashers of potential, active transformers, crucial interface, partnership

As long as there have been two or more people together on this planet, there has been the informal, but very real and essential activity of nursing, that is to say, the physical caring of one individual for another. Such care has been important for everyone from the delivering mother to the newborn and young child, to anyone one who has been injured, fallen prey to an illness, or grown old. It has known no geographical, demographic, or cultural boundaries. Nursing care is at the core of our humanity.

The word "nurse" is derived from the Latin *nutricia*, meaning "to nourish" or "to nurture." In a point to which we will return later, this Latin term is in contrast to the derivation of the word "physician," which has Greek roots in the word *physis*, with its clear relation to the physical (and less so the spiritual and emotional) world and the concepts of physiology and pathology. The concepts derived from these physical disciplines led to the interventions that today comprise the disciplines of medicine and nursing. The practice of medicine is not antithetical, but rather complementary, to the nourishing care of nursing; the distinction between the origins of the two arts is clear.

Consistent with the above perspective is Donahue's (2010) analysis of nursing as both the oldest of the arts and a young profession. For the Greeks, servants or slaves, both men and women, provided care for children and families. A millennium ago, deacons and deaconesses in Western churches provided nursing care to communities. From 500 to 1,400 CE (through the Dark and Middle Ages), knights, nuns, priests, and monks provided nursing care as the charitable acts required by their faith. Nursing flourished, while medicine was stagnant and without direction. With the advent of the Renaissance from the 1400s to the 1600s, medicine and science gained momentum, but nursing declined and remained in this state until the 1800s. Nursing care was poor during this period. Hospital nursing was staffed by convicts, widows, and orphans in exchange for food and shelter. In Asia, family members most often were the ones to provide nursing care.

Nursing as a formal and professional activity, with a larger and increasingly specific knowledge base, came into being with the work of Florence Nightingale. Born in 1820 to English parents in Italy, she attended the first nursing school, the Kaiserworth Deaconness Institute, in 1836. Her formal training was completed in only 3 months, but with that training, she and 38 other women went off to care for British troops in the Crimean War. With this group's efforts in hygiene, sanitation, and nursing practice, the death rate of injured soldiers dropped from 420 per 1,000 to 22 per 1,000. Nightingale's reforms and promotion of standardized nursing practice and formal education, along with her insistence that nurses show high moral character and high levels of technical skill, launched nursing as a true profession.

Following Nightingale was a long line of distinguished group of women who furthered the development of nursing as a respected and increasingly strong and important profession. In the United States, Clara Barton, Dorothea Dix, Linda Richards, Mary Mahoney, Annie Heeler, Isabel Robb, Lillian Wald, Mary Dutting, Clara Maass, Mildred Montag, Harriet Tubman, and Lucinda Ballard were among those who further developed the field. In 1873, the first professional nursing school in the United States was opened at Bellevue Hospital in New York City, and in 1888, in support of the concept that nursing was for men as well as women, the Mills Training School for Men was launched.

The profession of nursing has changed over the years since these early days. Today, there are Nurses Aides, Licensed Practical Nurses, Registered Nurses, Nurse Practitioners, and those with doctorates in nursing, with an increasing premium being placed on advanced nursing clinical practice, as well as research. In the latest effort to define the future of the field, its ability to meet the health challenges of the United States, and the needs of nursing for further development, the Institute of Medicine, in partnership with the Robert Wood Johnson Foundation, established a 2-year Initiative on the Future of Nursing. Specifically, this partnership established a committee whose charge was producing an action-oriented report containing recommendations for the future of nursing, including the educational and training needs, scope of practice, and policies at all levels of government that would enable the nursing profession to meet the demands of a U.S. health care system undergoing radical transformation (Institute of Medicine, 2010). More than this, the Committee considered what nursing can, and should be, for the future, that is, the next phase of the growth and redefinition of this critical profession that is so important to us all. What follows in this essay is my perspective on nursing and its future development.

MY INTRODUCTION TO NURSING

My first real introduction to nursing came during my general surgery internship and residency, and, even more, during my neurosurgical residency at what was then The New York Hospital and is now NewYork-Presbyterian Hospital and also at Massachusetts General Hospital and the National Institutes of Health Clinical Center in Bethesda, Maryland. Medical school education had not been as strong as one might have wished in many of the practical aspects of hospital care, and, at the time, interns and residents carried out a great many basic tasks, including drawing blood; inserting intravenous and intraarterial lines, Foley catheters, nasogastric tubes, drains and chest tubes; changing dressings and suturing wounds, and ordering bowel preps and enemas, as well as performing direct manual colon disimpactions and clean-outs in cases of severe constipation. All of this was in addition to performing all the other tasks of the young physician, from admission examinations and work-up orders to reviewing all the data collected for clearance for surgery, post-op follow-up, and even discharge, with appropriate rehabilitation and physical therapy orders. Of course, there was also the matter of providing coverage of patients on the floor and consults, as well as the myriad problems that could arise with patients on the general surgery and neurosurgical services. Patients on the latter service, in particular, were often quite ill; for example, with an intracranial bleed from a ruptured cerebral aneurysm or brain swelling after a craniotomy for tumor removal.

When problems arose late at night, and there was no senior resident or attending immediately available to help decide what needed to be done, it was the nurses who were always available to provide help. The help that the nurses provided was incredibly valuable and, most importantly, based on their familiarity with a given patient and the perspective provided by what was often long, practical experience. I quickly learned to turn to the nurses for advice and a solution to a given problem. For those late-night/early-morning calls, they could tell me that I needed to come see the patient or, often, that it was not really necessary. At the same time, they suggested what orders needed to be given to address the problem. There were times when I gave an order and the nurse involved would suggest that, perhaps, that was not the best thing to do. She would always provide an alternative suggestion or, if all else failed, a recommendation to call either the senior resident and/or the attending.

The training that the nurses provided was also invaluable. They were very much mentors to me and the other residents along the way. Their training went beyond the strictly medical to teaching ways to deal with family members and the various issues that often arose in association with the fears, hopes, and aspirations in situations with both serious and not-so-serious illness.

I cannot say enough about the team spirit and functioning that developed with nurses as time went on. This was true with both the surgical nurses and the floor nurses. As we worked more and more closely together, the mutual trust, respect, and camaraderie that we came to know not only provided for good patient care, but also made the time we worked together enjoyable. The nurses provided the core of that good experience. We came to celebrate good patient outcomes together and to share the pain when things did not go so well or we lost a patient. We came to teach each other and to care for each other.

The fact that the nurses spent much more time with both individual patients and their families than we as young physicians ever did (especially as we were often in the operating room all day), of course, meant that they always knew both patients and families better than we. However, it also became clear to me that the nurses were simply better attuned to, and more knowledgeable of, many such issues than we as physicians were ever likely to be.

I should add that, over the years since those days of residency, I have met and worked with many more nurses in some 32 countries around the world. Some, in resource-poor nations, struggle to provide optimal patient care amid great difficulties. They are heroic in their own right. Others fight to improve patient care and the position of nurses in developed countries. Despite the often-great economic differences, there are many common elements of struggle and achievement against daunting odds.

Among this large group of nurses, there are many outstanding leaders. Three nurses with whom I have worked closely over many years now include Dame Shelia Quinn and Shelagh Murphy, both very distinguished members of the Royal College of Nurses in the United Kingdom, and Pam Hoyt, RN, who is a colleague and leader at the Dreyfus Health Foundation (DHF). The work of these individuals around the world is outstanding, especially in relation to the DHF program known as Problem Solving for Better Health— Nursing®. Each of these individuals provides clear examples of what nurses can achieve. There is a fourth nurse of whom I am very proud and that is my daughter, Sara, whose pursuit of patient-centered research, as well as ever-better patient care, is exemplary.

When all is said and done, it is the special role of nurses as the direct interface with patients and families that has opened my eyes over time to the true nature of nursing and also the largely unrealized potential of nursing. It is that feature and further potential of nursing that I would like to explore in the rest of this chapter.

THE NATURE AND FUTURE OF NURSING

I believe that nurses and nursing are, and must be, the central point or organizing principle of any health care system. That has not been the traditional view. Rather, it has been the physician who has been presumed to be the center of the health care universe. Of course, physicians are partly to blame for this conception of the organization of health care, and the discipline as a whole has been resistant to giving nurses a larger and/or more important role. Additional factors, such as the level and rigor of education provided to, and/ or required of, nurses, and the historical domination of health care by males (physicians and administrators) in both the developed and developing worlds, have conspired to keep nursing in a subservient position. However, the organizational and economic structure of health care, as well as the demands placed on that structure, are changing. The result is that nursing can, and must, take a very central role in the new structure. The situation includes both significant challenges and opportunities.

Where do nurses fit into the structure of the health care system that is emerging? As Figure 20.1 shows, they are at the center

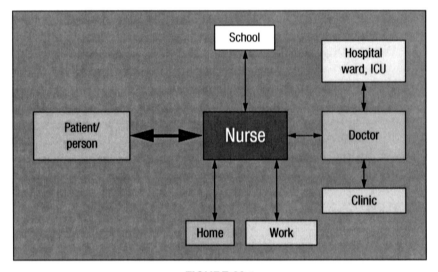

FIGURE 20.1
Nursing as the interface between people and health: Nurses as caregivers and facilitators.

as the interface between the physician and all other health care providers, as well as a host of other disciplines and the individual and family.

With this central role in mind, it is clear that nurses must be skilled, compassionate, and passionate professional caregivers; communicators and educators; health promoters; societal leaders and activists; as well as team members functioning in the real world. They are where the "rubber meets the road."

It is clear that the current structure of U.S. health care delivery—and that of many other countries—is failing to deliver the health care it should. The United States, which spends more on health than any other country in the world, that is, more than 14% of its gross national product (GNP), was only 37th out of 190 ranked health care systems around the world in 2000. Now, we know that there is much that is good about U.S. health care, but it simply is not achieving what it should or could. In addition, expenditures on health, whether in the United States or other countries, are rising rapidly and are unsustainable. To observe, as has been estimated, that at the current rate of increase the United States will be spending its entire GNP on health by 2050, makes clear just how serious the situation is and why a radical restructuring of the system is necessary. The situation does not have to reach a point anywhere near that extreme to create an untenable state.

While not denying that there are clear needs for specialized medical and nursing interventions and training, the fact is that health, in its broadest and most general sense, is a product of our society, that is, the larger world as well as the particular community in which we live. Although health care is moving in the direction of specialization by physiological system and/or disease state or type, human beings remain as integrated wholes, whose lives and quality of life cannot be so separated. Describing a person as a diabetic, or obese, or hypertensive does not begin to describe the whole person or predict or understand his or her behavior either within or outside the health care system. Doctors and nurse practitioners may prescribe a drug or therapeutic regimen, but follow-up to determine whether a prescription was ever filled, or the therapeutic regimen followed, is generally much less good. In fact, the very complexity of the health care system is unintentionally biased against successful therapy and, in some cases, leads to therapies for one system that compete, or interact negatively, with those for another problem prescribed by a different specialist. Confronted with such complexity and a system that most often communicates poorly within itself as well as with its clients, the individual with one or more health problems is left bewildered, often frightened, and even angry at a system that seems to make it difficult, if not impossible, for someone to secure the best care for himself or herself or a family member. Social workers, and even the new patient navigator (a new version of the previously operative ombudsman), can only do so much to help.

Quite beyond the complexity of the system is the fact that prevention of disease and health promotion are ultimately far more cost-effective and desirable than the treatment of a disease that could have been prevented. Health care cannot remain behind the walls of clinics or hospitals, but must move out into communities, where the most positive and cost-effective benefits, and the greatest good, can be achieved. This is where disease can be prevented or reduced in its intensity.

To move into the world where people live, raise families, and work, as well as contribute to the common good, one must understand that there are certain principles that are fundamental to the ultimate success of any such effort. The first tenet is that there is far too much unnecessary disease, suffering, and lost human potential secondary to disease and that this cannot be tolerated. The obvious correlate here is that every human life is of tremendous value, both intrinsically and in relation to its ability to contribute to the common good. The second principle is that a significant percentage of the disease burden of individuals and communities is secondary to human behavior and therefore subject to the positive effects of healthy lifestyle measures. Third is the fact that individuals and communities, given the proper education and tools, are going to be the most effective means of addressing the behaviors that lead to specific disease problems. Put another way, the people with the problems are not the problem. Rather, they are the solution, and their capacity to make the required changes must be unleashed. The fourth principle is that nurses and nursing are in the ideal position to act in the capacity of the unleashers of the potential of individuals and communities to take far more responsibility for their own health and for the healthy lifestyle and disease-prevention measures that are essential components of that responsibility. In effect, the individuals and communities must become an integral, active part of the health care system, rather than its (passive) objects.

Why are nurses and nursing so critical in the respect described above, as well as in health reform more generally? The answer has already been provided. They are the crucial interface between the complex, often highly technological health care system and individuals and communities. They have the ability to interact directly with individuals, families, and communities, as well as with the myriad of health care providers and payers, regulatory bodies, bureaucracies, and policy makers/legislators who are part of health care today, to achieve better health. A school nurse, for example, has contact not only with a child, but also with his or her family and the community at large because of the central place of any school in its community. A nurse who makes visits to homes gets to know patients and their families in ways that the physician never can. He or she can make a huge difference in the translation of a physician's or other clinic or hospital staff's orders (in the abstract) to something practical and effective because those orders and their necessity become reality and something to be carried out. The floor nurse in a hospital is the true interface with the patient and his or her family, again translating the physician's orders into practical terms and putting them into their proper place in the patient's world, however circumscribed that may be. The clinic nurse operates as the interface to the patient's and family's wider and real world, again educating, encouraging, and understanding the whole person, as well as the obstacles and challenges such a person faces every day both with respect to requisite treatment and the whole range of issues concerned with living. The nurse supervising individuals who may be serving their communities as community health workers of one sort or another is also their anchor, while the community people serve as his or her extension in the community to be certain that everyone is getting the best care possible and experiencing the highest quality of life attainable given the particular circumstances.

Can nurses do all these things? The answer is yes. I can state that without hesitation because of what I have seen nurses be capable of doing over the past 15 years as part of the Dreyfus Health Foundation's Problem-Solving for Better Health—Nursing (PSBH-N) program. Thousands of nurses in 32 countries around the world have participated and demonstrated the tremendous power within themselves to do so many different things. A dental nurse in Poland developed an oral health and anticavity program that became the national standard. A nurse in Fuzhou, China, trained another 1,000 nurses to be problem solvers, to be active transformers of the health care system there for the better. The list here is endless, but the proof is there. Details of many of the stories can be found in *Problem Solving Better Health: A Global Perspective* published by Springer Publishing Company in 2011. Among the many tools for enhancing nursing leadership, I believe that PSBH-N remains useful for building the future of nursing. It might be better to say that it can help unleash nursing's true potential.

The roles for nurses described above barely scratch the surface of what nurses and nursing can do, but they do provide a clear view of the critical role that nurses must occupy in the new health care delivery structure. I believe that nurses and nursing can, and must, seize the opportunity that is being presented for the good of people, as well as the good of the system. Nursing as a discipline is what will hold the new system together and make it function well.

Is the role for nursing that I have outlined compatible with the recommendations of the Institute of Medicine's 2010 report on *The Future of Nursing* cited at the beginning of this chapter? I believe it is. The Committee had four key recommendations:

- Nurses should practice to the full extent of their education and training.

- Nurses should achieve higher levels of education and training through an improved education system that promotes seamless academic progression.
- Nurses should be full partners, with physicians and other health care professionals, in redesigning health care in the United States.
- Effective workforce planning and policy making require better data collection and information infrastructure.

Of course, there is much more to each of these recommendations than can be discussed here. Without doing justice to the thought and evidence behind these broad goal statements, I would emphasize once again the centrality of nurses and nursing to health reform and the achievement of better health and quality of life for all the people. I would suggest that the statements of the Institute of Medicine/Robert Wood Johnson report could be augmented to reflect that point. Such a rendering could read as follows—as a kind of manifesto for the future of nursing.

The place of nurses and nursing as a discipline within the health care delivery system must be recognized as central, that is, the key interface between individual patients and their families and the entire health care system. Nurses are in the best position to improve the delivery of health care at the grassroots level and consequently to have the biggest cost-effective impact on individual, family, and community health because they act at this critical interface. The most important principle in this nursing effort is the enhancement of the capacity of individuals, families, and communities to take more responsibility for their own health, thus making them an integral and active part of the redesigned health care system The fact that there are 3,000,000 nurses in the United States alone emphasizes that this is an available workforce.

In accord with this, nursing should take a leading role in the redesign of the U.S. health care system, working closely and in partnership with physicians and other health care professionals. Although each professional discipline has its own important role, nursing principles will be used to define the core of the system. An important benefit of this redesign will be that physicians have more time to do what they do best, that is, diagnose and treat disease, develop new treatments and medicines, and contribute to the understanding of disease processes more generally.

Nurses should practice to the full extent of their education and training, with that training to include specific emphasis on the practical aspects of new models of health care delivery that incorporate individuals and families as integral and active components of that system. This means that nursing education and training will go well beyond the traditional subject areas to include integrated health care models, well-being and quality-of-life improvement tools, communication tools, family and community dynamics, understanding whole human lives, and outcome measurements.

Nurses should achieve higher levels of education and training through an improved education system that promotes seamless academic progression. However, that education must not be theoretical only, but rather incorporate major components of a practical nature such as those hinted at in the preceding paragraph. Such training and education should be goal directed, with the inclusion of outcome measures that demonstrate how the public has been better served by the added education and training. In other words, the higher levels of nursing education should ensure that nursing has a solid and central leadership role within the health care system. It must not only serve individual needs for career advancement, but also serve to build a new discipline with a new place in the overall system.

The advancement of nursing and nurses is crucial to the health of the people of the United States and many other countries. Nursing can, and should, be the beating heart of a health care system that both incorporates and serves the people and ensures an optimal quality of life for all.

The view of nursing put forward here is a radical one. Traditionally, medicine has been considered to be the essence of health care. Nurses and nursing have been handmaidens to this central figure. As important as medical care remains, however, health today must be seen in the far broader context of the total society. In fact, as stated earlier, the vast majority of "health" is a product of the functioning or malfunctioning of that society. Economics, education, the availability of jobs, recreation, faith, and a host of other things that make up people's lives and contribute to their total well-being, such as the need for compassion and respect, are part of that picture. Medicine in the form of physician-based care is not well positioned to bring all of these elements together to serve the best interests of the people and enable them to do more for themselves. Nursing is.

Of course, nursing cannot do everything, but, as the interface or pivot point of so many different factors and elements for individuals, families and communities, nursing can do much to ensure that the optimal health and well-being achievable is obtained for all people, while at the same time integrating those same people into the system as active participants. Although the challenges are daunting, the prospects for what can be achieved are exciting. Nurses and nursing need to seize the opportunity with which they have been presented for the sake of better health and life for all of us.

REFERENCES

Donahue, M.P. (2010). *Nursing, the finest art: An illustrated history* (3rd ed.). Maryland Heights, MO: Mosby Elsevier.

Institute of Medicine. (2010). *The future of nursing: Leading change, advancing health.* Washington, DC: National Academy of Sciences.

Smith, B.H., Fitzpatrick, J.J., & Hoyt-Hudson, P. (Eds.). (2011). *Problem solving for better health: A global perspective.* New York, NY: Springer Publishing Company.

Nurse Leadership in the Managed Care Setting

Derek van Amerongen

Commentary
by Joyce J. Fitzpatrick

Van Amerongen identifies the significant role of the nurse leader in managed care. According to him, the clinical background and expertise that the nurses bring provide an important competitive advantage. In addition to the clinical knowledge and skills, he identifies other important characteristics of successful nurse leaders, namely, sensitivity and empathy.

The Triple Aim of care, health, and cost serves as a framework for van Amerongen to discuss other key dimensions of leadership in managed care. These include being a culture-change agent, using knowledge of care systems, policies, and politics; developing an understanding of the care recipients as individuals first, rather than patients first; creating member-centric solutions within the managed care system; being data-driven; displaying a willingness to be measured; being comfortable with the virtual world, and being willing and ready to be part of a team.

Van Amerongen further describes the characteristic of leaders as inspiring others to do what he or she does, that is, "leading from the front." Sometimes nurse leaders describe their desire to clone themselves in order to accomplish the work that needs to be done.

*This understanding is consistent with the underlying
principle of inspiring others to be like them.*

*In his work, Van Amerongen has witnessed the
large impact that nurse leaders have had on millions
of individuals. He concludes that there are many
opportunities for more nurse leaders in managed care.*

Key focus areas: global view, culture-change agent, member-
centric, embrace innovation, lead from the front

I began my medical career as a practicing obstetrician in a very
busy community hospital in Chicago. Almost as soon as I began
my practice, I realized I was fascinated by the process of medical care
delivery: how it worked, or did not; how we served our patients, or
did not; and how all of the infrastructure that we typically took for
granted came to be. Over the next dozen years, I became more and
more involved in the administrative side of medical care. I wanted
to understand how to correct the many deficits of care that I saw
due to the problematic processes we used, but often never questioned. I wanted to understand medical delivery from a population
perspective as well as at the level of the individual patient. After
obtaining a master's degree in health administration, I moved to
the payer side at a large national insurer in order to be involved in
care management from a broader perspective. This move to a population focus entailed a change in my thinking. It made me view
the needs of patients—our health plan members—in a new light.
Just as I worked closely with nurses in the labor and delivery suite,
I continue to work closely with nurses in a different, but no less
important, capacity.

Perhaps the gravest challenges our medical care system
faces are how to improve quality, make the patient experience more
positive, and how to do so while moderating the exploding costs
of care. This has been called the Triple Aim, as elucidated by Don
Berwick of the Institute for Health Care Improvement and former administrator of Medicare. The work of the nurses in health
plans, both private and public (i.e., Medicare and Medicaid), is
critical to making these goals attainable. I learned very quickly of

the tremendous value that experienced and highly trained nurses bring to the interactions with plan members. It showed me a new dimension of the care delivery process and one that augments the care of the bedside nurse.

The care management nurse faces a different task than the nurse in the inpatient or outpatient setting. The focus for the latter is typically narrow: care for the patient during the acute treatment, then release the patient to home, a nursing facility, a step-down unit, and so on. The long-term outcome is really not the responsibility, or within the scope of care, of the hospital nurse. The same may be said of the nurse working in the traditional medical practice. Once the patient leaves the office, accountability for the patient's outcome diminishes. This is the turf of the care management nurse who is charged not only with making that transition successful, but also with overseeing the long-term status of the patient. This shift from an *episodic* to a *longitudinal* view is what care management is all about. It is highly valued by organizations involved in health maintenance. All too often the discussions about health focus solely on the negative: too much cost, too many complex patients, too many inappropriate services, and so on. Innovative organizations are realizing that successful clinical management can be a huge competitive advantage for both employers and health plans. Giving the right care at the right time can maximize the value of those services and avoid waste. Those companies that have healthier, more productive employees and beneficiaries will see better long-term outcomes than their competitors.

What are the hallmarks of a nurse leader in managed care? This shift in approach requires a particular kind of leadership. The basic skill set is similar to that of a nurse leader in any role. Certainly, we will always value sensitivity, empathy, clinical knowledge, and skills in a nurse professional. It is also fundamental that in the 21st century, every medical professional understands that *health is more than the absence of disease*. A global view of what creates health and improves quality of life, and what factors prevent that, is essential. However, there are some particular attributes that are highly valued for a nurse leader working with a managed population who seeks to bring to life the Triple Aim:

- Be a culture-change agent: Perhaps few skills are as important to the leader as being a promoter and facilitator of change. All medical care is in upheaval as we move through health care reform. This is actually a good thing, because we are being challenged to think in new ways and question the status quo. The leader must be prepared to create a positive environment for change to exist. Being open to new ideas, being a "glass half-full" person, and supporting team members who come forward with different approaches are all part of this evolution. At a strategic level, it is critical in this decade for leaders in any discipline of medicine to be knowledgeable about the rapid changes occurring in health policy and politics. The future of our profession is being determined even as we speak, mainly by forces outside of the medical establishment. Each of us needs to be conversant with what is driving that change, what it might mean, and how to make it work best for our patients and members. That means being aware of developments as they occur. Too many of my peers, both medical and nursing, are dissatisfied and unhappy about the current state of health care. I believe those feelings stem in large part from a failure to grasp what is happening in medicine and why. They feel powerless or sidelined. Knowledge is power, as well as a key to transforming change into positive results. Regardless of the feelings each of us may have toward the new environment of health care, it is here: we either step away, or engage it and make it work. This will often mean recognizing that without true change, we cannot get better. A transformative leader will be ready to educate staff and demonstrate through actions what kind of change is optimal. I have seen several nurse managers turn around departments that had lost their direction and were drifting without a real purpose. Pulling people together to achieve common goals that are clearly defined is hard work, but the culture that emerges will be powerful.

- Understand the individual is a person first, and a patient last: This reflects a different mindset than is traditionally seen in medicine. We are not usually taught to think about the person outside of the hospital or clinic. Although as patients we may want to be treated holistically, this is not the norm. Unfortunately, this ignores the reality that the individual faces. The time spent in the hospital is just one slice of a person's life. He or she is really not focused on the length of the inpatient stay. What he or she wants to know is more basic: What happens in a month? What level of activity can I perform? When can I go back to work? Does my spouse need to stay home to take care of me? Nurse leaders who instinctively understand those dilemmas are ones who guide their staff to proactively address those issues, and lay the groundwork for a successful transition to home. This gap between the traditional approach to medical care and what people actually need to have addressed was the impetus for embedding case management in what population-focused health plans do. One of my favorite examples is the case manager whose client was asked by the orthopedist to have biweekly follow-up visits post-op after a complicated hip procedure. The client's husband was elderly and not able to lift or drive the wife, yet he wanted to be there to hear the instructions and updates. The physician was unaware of the limitations of the couple to adhere to a rather demanding follow-up routine. His office was not trained or equipped to handle the logistics of this problem. This could have resulted in the member falling through a major crack, and blunting the ultimate benefit of the hip procedure. Understanding these family dynamics and limitations led the manager to find a free community-based shuttle that would pick up the couple, transport them to and from the office, and do so as often as the physician required. And it did so at no extra cost to the couple who were on a fixed income. This solution met their needs, as well as the physician's request. Viewing the individual in this way led to a true win–win result. This example also leads to the following key attribute:

- Create member-centric solutions: What are the options that are designed to make the *individual's* situation better, not necessarily that of the providers or the health plan? The endpoints to be met must be the member's. All too often the treatment goals, if spelled out at all, are only proxies for how the member feels or performs. For example, many hospital-developed discharge plans assess whether a member can walk from bed to bathroom. That is an important proxy for the ability to accomplish activities of daily living, but is not the complete answer to the question of whether a person is able to live independently once discharged to home. I learned this from a case manager who specialized in personally visiting the home of complex patients within the 48 hours after discharge. Seeing the actual home setting allowed her to understand more fully what the individual needed to be successful when coming home and to avoid a readmission. It took time, effort, and commitment to go beyond the standard discharge process, but it led to a dramatically better outcome. Good leaders understand this, and help their team deliver on member-centric care plans.

- Be data-driven: Remember that improving the quality of care is a key objective of the Triple Aim. Quality improvement cannot be done without quantifying what is done. The nurse leaders for the next decades must be comfortable with analyzing data of all sorts to identify new opportunities and to validate what is currently being done. For example, understanding the drivers of readmission requires tracking the frequency of specific diagnoses, the rates of unplanned admissions, the patterns of admissions across various hospitals, and so on. Using data allows us to lay the groundwork for future initiatives as the understanding of the drivers deepens. This is a core competency for the nurse leader managing a population who will be expected to bring new management ideas forward. One caveat is that this may pose an interesting dilemma for the nurse leader. As one delves into data, the results can sometimes initially look worse than expected. One large pediatric hospital enlisted our help in an intensive effort to delineate reasons behind asthma admissions. Some of the answers revealed quality problems in the hospital processes that were below the expected standards. But creating transparency even around the institutions' "warts" allowed it to dramatically improve the quality of asthma care and ultimately reduce unplanned admissions. The director of the project, a nurse working with our case management leadership, had the courage to stick with the decision to use data to guide change, even as the initial feedback was different than anticipated.
- Have the willingness to be measured: Having stressed the need to use and leverage data, health care professionals in the 21st century must be prepared to be measured and evaluated. Furthermore, we must be willing to have this information be completely transparent and public. I strongly believe that a basic reason so many people feel the health care system does not deliver value is that so much of what we do is hidden or not reported. Every hospital claims to give the best care; every practice claims to have the best doctors and nurses. What is the basis of these assertions? Typically, there is little that can be demonstrated to back them up. Consumers are increasingly demanding, and rightly so, they should be able to go online and compare one provider with another in objective, quantifiable ways. Nurse managers will be expected to measure and track performance of their staff, and be ready to have that data available for the world to see. This is

part of the culture change I referenced earlier. Making front-line nurses comfortable with this level of scrutiny will often be difficult, but it will be part of demonstrating that the organization is providing high-value care. These metrics need to be ones that are both meaningful and under the control of the nurses being reviewed. Our case management director created a dashboard for the case managers to track contacts, utilize statistics (including emergency room visits, admissions, etc.), and overall cost of care by diagnosis for the members they manage closely. The measurements were understandable to the team and viewed as meaningful trackers. The nurses can see their own progress and identify areas for improvement.

- Be comfortable with the virtual world: Few trends are as unsettling to experienced health care professionals over the past few years as the rapid evolution from actual to virtual interactions. This is a hard transition for those who learned their craft at the bedside. But this represents a deep-seated conversion that is remaking all industries, not just medicine. Many large corporations now expect a certain percentage of their employees will never physically sit in an office, but will work remotely. Aside from reducing overhead costs, it also permits greater flexibility of scheduling to meet the needs of the customer (remember: we are all about creating patient-centric solutions now!). Health plans have been leading this charge among health care organizations, but this is expanding across the entire industry. A few years ago, we made the decision that almost all of our nurses (over 700 nationally at the time) would work from home. The first year or two were very difficult. Few of us really appreciated what the change entailed. Criteria for the work-at-home environment had to be devised. Methods of communication that fostered high-quality interactions as well as support for the remote staff needed to be put in place. Tactics needed to be developed to bring people in many locations together as a team. Initially, in the early years, turnover was high and associate satisfaction was low. But since that time, our nurse leaders have become expert at linking a diverse group of professionals together into a high-performing team. Particular focus is given to promoting a sense of belonging and purpose. This strategic component is critical to complement the nuts-and-bolts issues of making sure the remote office functions are reliable and easy to use. Going forward, it is impossible to imagine placing a new individual into a leadership role who does not have a deep understanding of remote technology and the implications for nursing practice. Being adept at managing a virtual team has allowed us to offer care that better conforms to the member's schedule and needs, not ours. Interestingly, this has also become a relative competitive advantage for our organization in nurse recruitment. As people get more comfortable with the concept of telemedicine and remote work environments, many nurses, especially younger ones, seek us out as a potential employer. Despite the national nursing shortage, we are able to recruit effectively and fill vacancies promptly. This is a tribute to the skill and expertise of our nurse leaders who are able to identify the best candidates for our roles, and train them effectively.

- Be ready to be part of a team: We may look back on the first decade or two of the 21st century as the transition of medical care from an individual effort to a team approach. This may well be one of the most significant and long-lasting changes. Although we may have thought in the past that we worked as a clinical team, medical care has historically been very hierarchical, with a strict pecking order that rarely allowed for stepping out of traditional roles. Practitioners aside from physicians have not been encouraged to perform up to the limits of their professional expertise. This also means that the nurse leaders need to be prepared to support their staff in these activities, even if it disturbs the status quo. The team concept translates as identifying the clinical competencies of the staff members and leveraging those skills. It involves creating processes for hand-offs from one case manager to another that adds value to the case rather than detracts. We have nurses who specialize in various components of patient care: inpatient, catastrophic, home, obstetric, and so on. This specialization is acceptable as long as it does not lead to gaps in care, disruptions, or missed opportunities. Integration of data and systems and a deep understanding of the roles of each team member are hallmarks of a well-functioning unit. This cohesion is the primary responsibility of the nurse leader. The success of the team will be clearly demonstrated by the kind of data tracking described earlier. Additionally, working successfully with a team will increasingly mean working with nonclinical people. Our work around reducing readmissions, which is a major initiative for Centers for Medicare & Medicaid Services and health plans over the next few years, cannot proceed without cooperation with data analysts, social workers, hospital administrators, and so on. The need for close interaction with a variety of contributors will challenge the nurse leaders' team-building skills.

If I had to identify one trait that I expect all nurse leaders to have, it is that a leader inspires others to do what he or she does. I have seen this often in nurses who "lead from the front." Their ability and skill to take charge of situations and to work beyond the limits of a given scenario are so impressive that their peers gravitate to them for advice and direction. They want to emulate the behavior being modeled by the leaders who embrace innovation. They are not afraid of stepping out of the established patterns and trying novel approaches. In the 21st century, this is exactly what medical care needs to meet the needs and expectations of the public. We can no longer deliver mediocre care at enormous cost while consumers of medical services rightly complain about the lack of value they receive. But understanding the new model for nurse leadership in a managed population opens many avenues for achieving true health, not just delivering medical care.

For all of the negative perceptions of managed care, many of them justified, it has allowed nurse leaders an unparalleled opportunity to take on levels of decision making that are not options in the traditional care setting. I work with nurses who are involved in designing and implementing programs that will touch thousands and even millions of people. This can be a heavy responsibility, but it means nursing has established itself as a critical element of population health management in the health plan sphere. I believe nurse leadership will be essential to this transformation, and that the impact of nursing within managed care will only continue to grow. This sector of the medical industry is poised for explosive growth as population health management takes center stage in the era of health reform.

22

Advancing the Transformational Nurse Leader in an Optimal Health Care System

Steven A. Wartman

Commentary
by Joyce J. Fitzpatrick

*F*or Wartman, leadership is inspiration, grounded in teamwork and oriented toward achievement of shared goals. He shares with us his long history of working with nurses at many levels, from the bedside to the boardroom. Throughout his career, he has met successful and unsuccessful nurse leaders. He describes the successful nurse leaders as those who could defend their positions in a compelling and respectful manner. These were the nurse leaders who stood their ground, and who placed the patient at the center of their position or argument. This is an important message to nurse leaders everywhere.

Wartman provides key advice for potential and aspiring nurse leaders. He advises us to let go of the guild mentality, particularly important for nurses who aspire to leadership positions that transcend nursing. Furthermore, according to Wartman, nurses should be at the forefront of the efforts to change restrictive policies and regulations that hinder nurses and nursing. Nurse leaders are advised to become transformational rather than transactional leaders, and to move beyond the rewards and punishments inherent in transactional leadership styles. And importantly, the leader must learn that it is not all

about them, or as Wartman advises, taking the ego
out of the job.
   Wartman concludes with sage advice for
aspiring nurse leaders, beginning with developing
in-depth self-knowledge. He advises that aspiring
leaders seek career development experiences outside of
nursing. And throughout the entry, Wartman stresses
that leaders in health care should always put the
patient first.

Key focus areas: transformational, inspiring, compelling, confidence, self-awareness

I am an internist and sociologist who spent more than 25 years
in academic medicine, where I held a variety of leadership positions at several institutions (Residency Program Director, Division
Director and Professor of Medicine at Brown; Chairman of Medicine
and Director of Medical Services at Mount Sinai of Greater Miami
and Professor of Medicine at the University of Miami; Chairman
of Medicine and Physician-in-Chief at Long Island Jewish Medical
Center and Professor of Medicine at Albert Einstein College of
Medicine; and Dean of the School of Medicine, Executive Vice
President for Academic and Health Affairs, and Professor of
Medicine at the University of Texas Health Science Center at San
Antonio).

In 2005, I became the third president of the Association of
Academic Health Centers (AAHC), located in Washington, DC.
AAHC represents the part of a university that is usually led by a
Vice President for Health Affairs (or equivalent) and consists of
the health professions schools (medicine, nursing, dentistry, allied
health, pharmacy, public health, graduate studies, and veterinary
medicine), biomedical and clinical research programs, and the
owned or affiliated teaching hospital or health system. Our work
is a combination of member services (meetings and networking,
advocacy, consultation, published reports and issue briefs, and specific programs) and thought leadership (general trends, emerging

issues and challenges, and future directions). The Association has also been active globally with an international branch that was established in 2008.

On a personal note, I view myself as a "generalist and internationalist," with strong interests in and commitments to the development of policies, programs, and leadership that advance health and well-being through bringing academic programs in research and health professions education into better alignment with clinical programs that serve individuals and the community.

DEFINITION OF LEADERSHIP

Over the years, my definition of leadership has evolved considerably, from the traditional view of being a strong leader with a clear vision to one that encompasses being a transformational leader who inspires individuals and institutions to enhance and/or change their core values. In this regard, leadership is not so much a management or bureaucratic function, but a form of inspiration that combines individual and institutional respect with teamwork centered on mutual achievement.

PERSONAL EXPERIENCES WITH NURSE LEADERS

I have worked with nurses throughout most of my career. In a formative sense, these experiences began when, as a medical student at Johns Hopkins, I teamed intensively with home-visiting nurses in a study of differential rates of infant mortality in the former Yugoslavia. A critical part of the study involved home visits of newborn infants paired with visiting nurses. This experience was my initiation in gaining a deep understanding of the unique and important skill sets brought by nurses to the care of patients, where nurses impressively combined the social context of health with specific medical issues. A bit later on in my career, I worked with nurses when I was a Henry Luce Scholar in Indonesia, and learned a great deal from the way nurses were able to skillfully integrate traditional Indonesian medicine with Western medicine. Bridging this gap illustrated for me the profound ability of nurses to prioritize the interests of patients in the context of any particular scientific or other belief system.

I brought this spirit with me to my first academic position at Brown University and Rhode Island Hospital, where I practiced side by side with nurses in the general medicine clinic, the emergency room, and other areas. When we created a new residency program in general internal medicine, nurses were part of the program's development and implementation team. As a result, the residents gained meaningful team experiences in a variety of settings.

As I moved up the academic ladder, I increasingly interacted with nurses in senior leadership positions: hospital and health system nurse leaders, nursing deans, and nurse leaders in a variety of associations and organizations. At this level, I began to understand why some nurse leaders were more successful than others. The more successful nurse leaders were able to describe and, if necessary, defend their positions in a manner that was respectful but compelling. They did not back down easily, but they were able to acknowledge when someone had a better idea. They always managed to put the welfare of the patient at the center of their approach or argument, and they were not daunted by those physicians who tended to either disregard or disparage their ideas. On the other hand, the least successful nurse leaders seemed incapable of articulating their positions forcefully or compellingly; they hesitated to take the lead on issues and consistently deferred to physician leadership even when their positions were fundamentally sound.

LESSONS LEARNED

Nurses have important and vital leadership roles to play in all aspects of the health system. Their perspectives are invaluable in bridging the gap between the technical experience of health care and its meaning in the lives of patients and their families. In order to provide the most effective and "transformational" leadership, potential nurse leaders should focus their efforts on four areas:

1. **Eliminate the "guild mentality."**
   Nursing, like the other health professions, has a rich and deep history that exemplifies the creation of a guild, in which members share a particular set of values and beliefs. Guild members believe that they are "special" because they have unique qualifications that differentiate themselves from others not in the guild. Although some form of group identification is normal

and can have its positive qualities in any profession, in nursing it may be particularly inhibiting to those who aspire to leadership positions that transcend the field of nursing.

2. **Change restrictive policies and regulations that weaken the role of nursing.**
   Whether it is state licensing requirements, scope-of-practice laws, or university policies and procedures, nurse leaders need to be at the forefront of the movement to change these policies and regulations with an eye toward improving the care of patients. It is critical that practitioners are able to practice up to the full scope of their capabilities. Similarly, it is important that the numerous arrays of regulations impacting the health professions are better "harmonized" so as to permit the most effective approaches to team care.

3. **Seek to become a "transformational" as opposed to a "transactional" leader.**
   Transactional leaders lead by a system of reward and punishment. Although sometimes necessary, I believe that this approach is often short-sighted and does not always achieve good long-term results. Transformational leaders, on the other hand, seek to change institutional culture by instilling and inspiring core values and beliefs within the organization. This kind of leadership requires the ability to have:
   - *Idealized influence* in order to espouse an institutional vision with energy, determination, and focus;
   - *Inspirational motivation* to confidently and effectively communicate one's vision and guiding principles;
   - *Intellectual stimulation* to challenge others to work together to find new or innovative solutions;
   - *Individualized consideration* that recognizes the contributions of others as well as others' goals and aspirations; and
   - *Intercollegial consideration* in which one works to harmonize the diversity of agendas and issues that arise in complex organizations.

   As nurses explore more openings to become leaders in our health care system, they are poised to use these opportunities to become exemplars of transformational leadership. (Antonakis, Avolio, & Sivasubramaniam, 2003; Bass, 1999, 2008)

4. **Learn to take the ego out of the job.**
   A substantive issue regarding effective leadership is whether the job is all about the individual or the organization. Strong

leaders who impress others with charisma and good speaking skills, although appealing, may be more interested in promoting themselves than the institution. In general, leaders who are unable to take the ego out of the job, or, as it is commonly expressed, "to bask in the reflected glow of others," often fail as transformational leaders in being able to change organizational culture. I believe the most effective leaders place the needs and aspirations of their institutions ahead of themselves, something that requires considerable confidence and self-awareness.

AN EXAMPLE OF TRANSFORMATIONAL NURSE LEADERSHIP

A number of years ago, I was part of a hospital-based team that was charged with the development of "critical pathways" for some of the more commonly admitted inpatient diagnoses. As the pathways were being created, we were following the approach of offering the admitting physician the option of using the pathway instead of writing an individualized order set. At an important point in the discussion, a nurse leader jumped in with the idea that, rather than make the critical pathway an "option" for the admitting physician, the critical pathway be designed as the "default" option, so that the physician would have to consciously make the decision to write a separate order set. This proposal was initially met with a negative reaction, mostly based on the idea that physicians do not like to be told what to do and don't want to practice "cookbook" medicine. The nurse leader calmly heard the feedback and then eloquently pointed out that our most important objective is the improvement of patient care and that it would be beneficial to also improve the physician experience at the same time. She suggested as the next steps that we review the literature on physician behavior and sample a group of physicians to get their opinions. The literature review found many interesting ideas and concepts and the group of physicians sampled mostly approved the idea—they saw it as making their work somewhat easier while giving them the option to individualize care as needed. The nurse leader was careful not to be either authoritarian or inflexible, but rather came across consistently as having the best interests of both patients and physicians in mind. Rather than appearing to own the idea, she worked tirelessly to enlist the support and cooperation of others so that her idea became everyone's idea. She was, in short, a transformational leader.

RECOMMENDATIONS FOR ASPIRING NURSE LEADERS

Those who aspire to any leadership position, regardless of background, need to have an in-depth understanding of themselves. They need to be able to realistically assess their strengths and weaknesses, and to use these insights to develop a strong and effective leadership team. For nurses in particular, transformational leadership is especially challenging, given the traditional hierarchies in the medical fields and academia. I would urge aspiring nurse leaders to think broadly, learn from the best and worse characteristics of leaders around them, and—always—put the patient first in decision making wherever possible. Career development pathways certainly vary, but I would suggest that leadership include positions outside of nursing at some point in order to gain important perspective and experience. But most of all, leaders need to look carefully within themselves and develop the confidence, based on a set of principles of their own devising, to inspire others to work toward a common set of goals.

REFERENCES

Bass, B. M. (1999). Two decades of research and development in transformational leadership. *European Journal of Work and Organizational Psychology, 8*(1), 9–2.

Bass, B. M. (2008). *The Bass handbook of leadership: Theory, research and managerial applications* (4th ed.). New York, NY: Free Press.

Antonakis, J., Avolio, B. J., & Sivasubramaniam, N. (2003). Context and leadership: An examination of the nine-factor full-range leadership theory using the Multifactor Leadership Questionnaire. *Leadership Quarterly, 14*(3), 261–295.

Nursing Leadership: A Perspective From a Friend of Nursing

Louise Woerner

Commentary
by Joyce J. Fitzpatrick

*W*oerner describes herself as a friend of nursing; she has participated as a leader for many years in many nursing forums. In fact she says she is in awe of nurses. Although the large successful business she created is a home care service, providing nursing and other health care services to thousands, she did not purposely set out to become so connected to the nursing world. But she identified an unmet need, and put her knowledge and business acumen to work.

Woerner believes that leaders, by definition, must have followers. Further, leaders must provide their followers with a clear direction. In addition, there are several other core competencies of leadership that Woerner describes, including good communication, ability to make the tough and often unpopular decisions, resilience, self-knowledge, and risk taking. Accordingly, the visionary leader looks ahead, often requiring the followers to take a leap of faith to follow.

According to Woerner, nurse leaders must be able to understand various perspectives. An extremely important point made by Woerner in relation to nurses is that often the support is not available from within, especially for women in leadership roles in nursing. If this is the case, as Woerner's experiences and observations suggest, it is an extremely important issue for

> *nurse leaders to address. Positive regard within the ranks of nursing is key to the future of the profession of nursing, and the preparation of future leaders. As an exemplary health care leader, Woerner shares lessons learned, including learning from mistakes and that success often requires a strategy adjustment.*

Key focus areas: self-knowledge, self-renewal, followership, failing forward, collaborate

I have often been called a friend of nursing. From my perspective, I am an admirer of nursing and nurses. In fact, I am virtually in awe of nurses. I became part of the health care system through a turn in my business concept based on the regulatory environment in New York, and through that, an admirer of nurses. I was working as a consultant in Washington in the 1970s as an analyst, looking at the implications to Social Security as the population aged, as women moved into the workforce, and families become more mobile. This data led me to wonder who would provide homemaker services such as meal preparation, assistance with bathing and dressing, to individuals who wished to live independently in their own homes. I thought there might be an opportunity to provide the "services" women used to perform when they were at home to do them and when families lived closer together.

Having immersed myself in demographic facts and statistics, I needed to determine whether there would be a market for these services. I thought of my early experience as a 5-year-old "hospice worker," caring for my grandmother who died in our home of breast cancer. Later in life, after the early death of my mother, I was faced with my father's request that I return home to live and care for him. My dad was from the generation of men who thought that socks came out of the drawer and milk came out of the refrigerator. I was willing to help, but the thought of moving back home to help my dad so early in my career, for which I had prepared by working my way through the completion of master's degree in business administration from the University of Chicago, was less than appealing.

But I struggled to find services I could purchase so my father could live independently. I could not find them. The essence of a business emerged: an unmet need, which fit my concept of a viable business. Businesses must provide something people want. Most people do not want to go into a nursing home. They would prefer to stay independent with services in their homes. The concept, based in home economics, was to develop such a service.

I went back to Rochester to start HCR several years later, and became part of the health care delivery system because in New York, providing home care services requires a doctor's order with nursing supervision. Aides who work in people's homes had to complete a New York State-approved training program, and be supervised by a nurse. There were more complex regulations than I had envisioned, but this was New York. So began my work with nurses, which is interesting as I had worked hard to have a career choice other than the traditional one of nurse, teacher, or secretary.

Today, I am proud to say, HCR is a thriving certified home health care agency with over 950 employees and locations in nine counties across New York State. HCR has been consistently recognized as a leader in home health care. HomeCare Elite placed HCR in the top 500 of the approximately 10,400 certified home health agencies in the United States. HCR is one of only 42 agencies that have been in the top 500 all 5 years of the award. We have achieved this status because of the commitment, caring, and leadership of our nurses. Additionally, HCR was awarded the Rochester Business Ethics Award for large companies, also a reflection of the integrity of nurses, the most respected members of the health care profession.

I became even more interested in nursing leadership as I entered the national nursing scene when friends from the women's movement, and members of the Zonta Club of Washington, DC, identified me as a candidate for the National Advisory Council on the NIH Center for Nursing Research. Through that appointment, I met extraordinary nurse scientists and leaders and had the opportunity, with the support of nurse leader, Colleen Conway-Welch, PhD, RN, CNM, FAAN, FACNM, Dean and Professor at Vanderbilt University's School of Nursing, and others, to found the Friends of the National Institute of Nursing Research, and serve as the organization's founding president. I have also had the honor of serving 12 years on the National Advisory Committee for the Robert Wood Johnson (RWJ) Executive Nurse Fellows Program. Through these experiences, I have had the privilege of working with many of the country's brightest nurse leaders, which has only deepened my passion and admiration for nurses and the field of nursing. That experience forms the basis for my comments in this chapter.

DEFINITION OF LEADERSHIP

Richard Beckhard defines leadership as a relationship between leaders and followers. To expand on that definition, it is important to note that I believe that to be a leader, one must have followers. Quoting President Dwight D. Eisenhower, "Leadership is simply the art of getting someone else to do something you want done because he/she wants to do it." You need a relationship with those followers based on actions that match the rhetoric. You need energy to support and nurture followers as well as to achieve your goals.

Over the course of my career, I have come to know there are many different types of nurse leaders. Leadership has to incorporate some flexibility based on the situation and the goal. For instance, a generally practiced collaborative style of leadership may need to be adjusted to a "command and control" model in an urgent situation. So instead of "defining" leadership, I prefer to think of leaders in terms of core competencies.

Effective leaders must be good communicators, as communication is a core leadership trait. Today, the complexity of forms of communication present a mastery challenge for the leader who must have expertise and abilities in written, oral, electronic, and digital forms of communication and able to use both visual strategies and language.

Leaders must be good at establishing a clear direction and providing followers with information so they can make accurate and informed decisions. Followers need to have a feedback loop, so a leader's listening skills must be sharp. When followers are well informed and supported, they gain confidence that there is progress toward the leader's direction or vision.

Along with communication, effective leaders must be able to make the tough and often unpopular decision, which is sometimes referred to as managerial courage. It is important to lead from the front of the issues based on principles, vision, and mission. Leaders who have this ability will let people know where they stand, give both positive and corrective feedback to others, deal with situations quickly and directly, and are not afraid to take action when necessary—popular or not—as a necessity to progress toward a goal or vision. When leaders step forward courageously with their followers, they must be careful not to seem overly critical or heavy-handed when addressing issues, because followers may not find the courage to proceed as easily as the leader.

One of the key leadership qualities of focus in the Robert Wood Johnson Executive Nurse Leaders Program is self-knowledge. Knowing and recognizing one's personal strengths, weaknesses, and limits, seeking feedback from others, and gaining insight from mistakes can allow even the most successful, seasoned leader to grow. Additionally, it is important for the intense and passionate leaders to have enough self-knowledge to see how they are reflected in the eyes of others, and make adjustments to communicate their expectations, which may not be the same for others as they are for themselves. In thinking of one's self, it is always helpful to have a sense of humor about one's frailties. Leaders who can use self-deprecating humor and laugh at themselves allow their followers room to be kind to themselves and to have fun as they work toward a vision or goal.

Risk taking is a quality leaders need. This is a challenge for many nurses, who have not been educated in how to calculate risks. What many nurses see as a risk would not be thought of as risk taking to most. As nurse leaders emerge and develop, thinking about their risk profile is very beneficial. Leaders do not take crazy risks. They evaluate situations and often need to proceed with less than complete certainty of how things will play out. When a risk produces a negative result, quick action and correction is required. I call this failing forward and will expand on that later.

Visionary leaders are going where no one has gone before. They look ahead, take trends from the ether. These futurists are scary to some individuals who cannot put together seemingly unrelated ideas, trends, and facts into the same vision as the leader. The leap of faith behind such a leader can be based on past experience, loyalty, or other factors leaders are able to instill.

As part of the National Advisory Council for the RWJ Executive Nurse Fellows Program, there were two leadership concepts discussed about which I disagree: balance and servant leadership.

Self-renewal is critical for leaders and different from balance. Most leaders I have known do not enjoy a balanced life. They are driven by their goals and/or their passion. Most of their energy and thinking is focused on their objective and their followers. Accomplishing great things often takes sacrifice, or is achieved at the expense of something else. I never agreed that leaders could live, or even should aspire to live, a balanced life. At the same time, I do agree that intensity and passion taken to an extreme can be off-putting, rather than motivational or inspirational. Very intense and passionate leaders can be intimidating to followers, who do not aspire to the level of commitment they see in very intense and passionate leaders. The problem about balance is that the leaders cannot schedule their timing of the demands of progress toward their goals, or the needs of followers. At the same time, when there is opportunity, leaders must engage in self-renewal. It is important for a leader to know how to recreate, that's why they call it recreation.

At RWJ's Executive Nurse Fellows Program, one of the last sessions before conclusion of the program and a frequent topic of discussion among alumni of the program is leadership renewal. There is a need for both self-renewal and for organizational renewal. This was discussed by John W. Gardner in his 1981 book *Self-Renewal*. The concern for renewal has to focus on the rapidly moving health care environment. Individuals cannot afford to get stale or burned out. Organizations must engage in a continuous process of assessment and strategic redesign in order to stay effective, vital, and relevant.

It has been my observation that the concept of a servant leader resonates among nurses. Even after reading and discussing this concept, I really do not believe that there is such a person. By definition, I do not think that a servant can be a leader. Although I agree that you can lead in many ways other than by positional power, and although I agree with many of the "powers of the weak," I still think that the servant leader concept plays into the weaknesses of nurses who want to be leaders, but do not want to take risks, fail forward, take chances, and simply stand up when necessary. It seems to me that the concept mistakes the leader/ follower relationship, which is key to achieving a goal or vision.

The leadership styles I admire the most are those that are positive and optimistic. I do not believe that you can lead people based on fear, because as soon as the feared event or reality occurs, those individuals will no longer follow. There is also the pied piper type leader, who is fun based. Those leaders are exciting and fun to be around.

EXPERIENCE WITH NURSE LEADERS

Nurse leaders have a particular leadership challenge, perhaps not different from the challenges of many others, but it seems to be more of an obstacle in nursing: the need for positive feedback, the need to be liked (vs. simply respected). One of the motivations of going into nursing is to provide positives for others and to receive the positives back. This goal cannot always be achieved as leaders develop.

Leaders have to be able to take some negatives, especially when pushing through the changing times health care faces today. Many leaders are loved, and that works well for nurse leaders, but others are simply admired or respected, and may not "feel the love," which some nurse leaders have indicated to me is important. The challenge is to focus on the vision and be able to take some of the "cold pricklies" that are interspersed with the "warm fuzzies" when bringing about change.

Nursing is a caring profession, so one cannot expect nurse leaders to drop the caring and become cut-throat leaders. However, nurse leaders do need to learn not to take situations with other followers and other partners too personally. For instance, as health care is changing, former competitors may become partners, and former partners may become competitors. The leaders must not personalize these changes. Nurse leaders must use their valuable assessment skills to great advantage and be nimble. Lifelong learning is an element of agility that is a great strength of the health care leaders of today. In New York, there is no continuing education requirement for nurses. I hope this does not imply that lifelong learning is optional.

The worst leaders control and manipulate information. As a result, they can miss key and valuable information in a feedback loop that might benefit their decision process, because others whom they lead do not have the full picture. Today, particularly, people expect transparency. Other bad leaders fear other experts and collaborators or partners. As a result, they may not maximize results. According to Ducker (2001), if you can't collaborate, you'll be gone.

LESSONS LEARNED

One of the most important concepts or lessons that I have learned is that good leaders learn from failure. "Failing forward" is a concept in our organization. When something does not work, approach the goal differently. When a leader is moving into uncharted territory, risk is inherent. Thinking about risk taking brings one to the issue of failure. I have "failed forward" in my career. The point is that failure is usually part of moving ahead. Success often requires an adjustment in strategy and/or tactics, as one avenue fails to produce the desired result. This type of failure may be characterized as a lesson learned. As scientists know, often finding out what something is not is a key step in finding out what something is.

Early in my career, I adopted a personal philosophy that the people doing the work know the most about the work. This is supported as a case in point, a lesson I learned. As you can imagine, transportation is an essential factor in providing home care. My management team struggled with how to get more workers with cars or how to provide transportation for our workforce, particularly our home health aides. Public transportation was not really a viable option, and still isn't, especially as hours provided to individuals have become shorter. Our leadership team came up with various ideas like buying a taxi company. When I finally took this issue to our Home Health Aide Advisory Committee, one of the home health aides said, "Geez Looouise, why don't you help us get driver's licenses and cars? It will be better for everyone." That idea was such an elegant solution to a critical issue. HCR began a successful "Roadway to Independence" program that took our home health aide employees from "bussers" to car owners, which enabled more care to be delivered in the hard-to-reach suburbs, and offered a new opportunity for both our patients and employees. Leaders need to be good listeners, particularly to the people doing the work. This presents a great opportunity for nurse leaders, as nurses are recognized as the members of the health care team who know the most about the work of caring for patients.

Listening well can help resolve any leadership issue. When you can find the answer in yourself as a leader, you can find it in your followers. Smart leaders in health care reform will look to nurses. This provides a followership opportunity for nurses in addition to the leadership roles.

IMPLICATIONS FOR LEADERS WITHIN NURSING

Leaders can listen and understand issues from more than one perspective. Advocacy for patients is an important role for nurses, but it is not sufficient to be a nurse leader. To advocate, one must be able to marshal arguments. Data and ideas provide a strong basis for a leader's position. When leaders want to press for a position, the advocacy or arguments need to be posed within a context that resonates with other leaders or decision makers in the organization. Nurses who want to be leaders in the redesign of the health care system need to understand the challenges from the various perspectives and to be able to make their points within the context of the organization and its mission, or within the policy direction.

An observation about nurse leaders, which is often written about, is that they don't always get the support and encouragement they need from other nurses. It is important to have colleagues who can say, "You go, girlfriend." Male nurse leaders seem to need less of this support, or maybe the expectations for how they lead are different from those for other nurses. I see this as a major concern for the field. If nursing is to develop leaders, it is important for other nurses to support them, especially to others in health care. I would even suggest that you might not necessarily agree or understand where a nurse leader you observe is going, but staying on a positive note about that person can help assure that there are more nurse leaders. Each time a nurse leader is diminished, it affects other nurse leaders. Unfortunately, stereotypes can take on a sense of reality, and when nurses are not supported, it becomes all too easy to generalize to the lack of leadership in the field.

A variant of this point is that leadership is not a zero sum game. Leaders who support others create a larger whole. In addition, as Ronald Reagan said, "There is no limit to what can be accomplished if it doesn't matter who gets the credit." Versions of this quote are attributed to Emerson, Truman, John Wooden, and even former LDS Church President Harold B. Lee.

CONCLUDING THOUGHTS

Benjamin Disraeli advocated "constancy to purpose." That trait of perseverance is a key element of success. Leaders must also be resilient. Success is often measured in steps taken forward, after some steps are taken backward. Success does not usually follow a straight upward trajectory, so it is very important for leaders to stay optimistic, to be able to take setbacks in stride but keep constant to the goal. Home care is a nursing-driven business with quiet leaders. Our industry is looking for more highly visible nurse leaders, who can advance the role of home care within the health care delivery system. Today, we have too few at the table to assure the value of our small component of the delivery system is understood and funded. Who will be those leaders?

REFERENCE

Drucker, P. (2001). *The essential Drucker: The best of sixty years of Peter Drucker's essential writings on management.* New York, NY: Harper Collins.

Gardner, J. W. (1981). *Self-renewal: The individual and the innovative society (rev.ed.).* New York, NY: W. W. Norton.

Closing Thoughts on Nursing Leadership From the Present Into the Future: Perspectives From a Collaborative Team

Victor J. Dzau and Catherine L. Gilliss

Following the release of the Institute of Medicine (IOM) Report, *The Future of Nursing: Leading Change, Advancing Health* (IOM, 2011), significant attention has focused on each of the report's eight recommendations. Two of the recommendations are especially salient to the issue of nursing leadership:

Recommendation 2: Expand opportunities for nurses to lead and diffuse collaborative improvements; and

Recommendation 7: Prepare and enable nurses to lead change to advance health.

In response, professional organizations, such as the North Carolina Nurses Association, have developed the Leadership Academy for early–mid career aspiring leaders. The Johnson and Johnson Foundation has launched its Developing Advanced Practice Nurses as Leaders in Clinical Settings program. The national focus on nursing leadership has sharpened.

This volume has addressed an influential aspect of leadership in nursing—how it is perceived by others. In leadership, the perspectives of others matter. Because success in leading partially results from matching the leader's activities to the expectations of those who would be led, leaders must explore what is expected of them as well as how they are perceived. *How nurses are perceived as leaders by those outside the nursing* profession informs the practice of leadership in nursing.

Leadership represents many things to many people but, importantly, the *perception* of leadership and matching the leadership behaviors to the *expected or desired* behaviors is a powerful contributor to whether or not leadership is successful. Leaders need to know what those whom they are leading expect from the leader. In the general case of nursing, the expectation set of others is complex.

The term "nurse" represents a wide range of roles, work experiences, and educational levels. The woman wearing a white smock greeting patients in the physician's office is a "nurse," although she may not actually hold any credential that would legally title her as a "nurse." The doctorally prepared, funded professor is a "nurse," as is the doctorally prepared Chief Nursing Officer. That nurses have been portrayed in stereotypic ways in the media contributes to a wide social misunderstanding of the work of the nurse, and the fact that much of nursing's work is knowledge work renders it invisible and difficult to convey to the public.

Within the health care team, contacts between physicians and nurses occurring early in the training or work experience form an imprint. Nurses can be viewed as knowledgeable and supportive or difficult and dull. Although some physicians instruct those beginning their medical careers to take advice from nurses, others will convey the impression that if nurses were so smart they should have gone to medical school. Both of these positions are stereotypes that can delay the development of strong professional alliances.

Annual reports by Gallup consistently report the public view that nurses are "the most trusted professionals." Although trusted, *are nurses seen as leaders*? The previous chapters offer insights into the views of others. We offer our closing thoughts on this subject through the lens of collaborators who work in an academic health system in which nurses hold key positions within the leadership structure and an accompanying level of respect for their leadership. Using our own work environment, we will describe the leadership qualities and accomplishments of a few of our nurse colleagues in leadership positions. From these brief descriptions, we will offer some generalizations on why we believe they have been successful in their leadership positions. In closing we will offer our view of a preferred future in health care and explain why we believe nursing leadership will be so critically important to effecting the needed changes in health care.

THE PICTURE OF NURSING LEADERSHIP AT DUKE

Duke University Hospital (DUH), the flagship hospital of the Duke University Health System (DUHS), is a 924-bed tertiary care facility, and Kevin Sowers, MSN, RN, FAAN, serves as its president. Prior to his appointment as president, Kevin served as the hospital's chief operating officer. His career in nursing began as a staff nurse in oncology, and he "worked his way up." You cannot walk the halls of Duke Hospital without realizing that everyone knows him and would like to speak with him. He is socially poised, always attentive to details about people and the environment, and always willing to stop to talk with a patient or his or her family member to ask, "How are we doing?" "Anything I need to know to make your stay better?" "Anything I can do for you?" He knows the staff and inquires about their family members. He speaks with everyone while continuing to move through the hospital. A man on a mission. Kevin Sowers is a nurse who leads a complex organization.

Kevin has the professional background of a nurse and always acknowledges that he is a nurse, but he uses his talents to solve problems on behalf of the patients served by Duke Hospital and the full range of staff Duke Hospital employs. His focus is on the good of the whole. He seeks input from many corners of the organization and maintains an interdisciplinary perspective.

Kevin knows what is expected of him. He prepares for meetings and stays focused on the work while working; he does not waste the time of his colleagues. He is clinically knowledgeable across a wide range of topics from direct patient care issues to the business practices that support patient care. His colleagues trust him and he gets results.

Recently, Duke opened a new Duke Cancer Center. Kevin was very much engaged in the design process and detailed aesthetics, from the fireplace in the entryway to the piano in the atrium. As with other parts of his work, he is connected to the architectural details as well as the larger issues, including use of light and space. He brought the point of view of the clinician to this building project and connected it to the point of view of the cancer patient.

During this time of dynamic change in the health sector, strategy requires innovation, and effective innovation requires managing change. Anna Lore, BSN, Assistant Vice President for Health System Innovation Planning, is a master at walking people through needed change. Anna has been described as the person who connects others, convening groups of people who may not know one another but who should work together to advance an organizational goal.

Anna's career has included administrative experience in managed care organizations as well as time in government affairs. As a consequence, she has a broad perspective integrating organizational priorities and dynamics with institutional and public policy. The breadth of her experience sets her up as a likely convener. Her skilled communication work, particularly at briefing executives and coaching others where they are needed in any project, facilitates the process for groups working on novel issues.

Although most people know Karen Frush, MD, as a pediatrician and the chief patient safety officer for the DUHS, she often introduces herself as nurse-doctor. Karen completed a bachelor of science in nursing (BSN) before entering medicine, and that is a point of pride for her. She is viewed as an advocate for best practices and for outcomes that benefit the patient. Karen is a master trainer for the U.S. Department of Defense TeamSTEPPS (Team Strategies & Tools to Enhance Performance & Patient Safety) program. She introduced TeamSTEPPS into the health system and is widely recognized as an advocate for all. Generally appearing to be low-key and widely understood to be a good listener, Karen does not get caught up in energy-zapping exchanges that serve no common good. Although busy, she focuses on the details that matter to accomplish her goals, and she accomplishes a great deal. She is well respected, and her opinions are sought by members of the health care team from all disciplines. A member of the DUHS Executive Management Committee, she is the go-to person for thinking through complex problems, many of which are interdisciplinary in nature. She often comments that she learned the skills she relies upon to accomplish her goals in her basic nursing education.

Mary Ann Fuchs, DNP, RN, FAAN, serves as the Vice President of Patient Care and System Chief Executive in the DUHS. Her successful career in leadership began at DUH, where she worked as a staff nurse in oncology. She took on progressively more complex leadership challenges and became the chief nursing officer of the hospital system in 2000. Meanwhile, she completed a Wharton leadership program and was selected into the Robert Wood Johnson Executive Nurse Fellows Program. She completed her doctor of nursing practice (DNP) degree while continuing to work full time as a busy executive leader. Mary Ann knows how to manage many things at once.

When she began her system leadership role, she was responsible for the nursing and patient care services staff in three hospitals and the related clinics and ambulatory services. Although enfranchised as a single health system, the various entities were not aligned. The nursing staff did not know each other across the entities and no one was quite sure their own entity would benefit from a common mission, vision, or values statement. Mary Ann developed a thoughtful and comprehensive strategic plan that helped them understand why that needed to change and helped them accomplish the change so successfully that within 6 years, they were aligned, working regularly together, and each of the three hospitals had achieved American Nurses Credentialing Center Magnet Recognition.

How did she lead over 6,000 nurses toward these accomplishments? She convened them. She listened to them. She encouraged them to lead one another. And she represented their work effectively to the other executive leaders in the health system.

When she returned to her alma mater as dean and professor at the Duke University School of Nursing, Catherine Gilliss, PhD, RN, FAAN, entered an academic health center poised for change. The president of the university had been in place for 3 months. Her immediate supervisor, the Chancellor for Health Affairs, was also new to the university. Catherine's experience as a dean at another university prepared her to see the opportunities at Duke for someone willing to work hard toward making a difference (coincidentally, the university's first strategic plan following her appointment was titled "Making a Difference").

In accepting the appointment at Duke, Catherine worked to make the case that the School of Nursing, including its programs, faculty, staff, and students, could play a larger role in the academic health center and in the university. She proposed a vision for the School to the chancellor and explained how to make that happen. She made the case for resources that she believed would bring a return on investment. Believing in the fundamental need for strong respect and cooperation between nursing education and nursing service, she sought and was awarded the title Vice Chancellor for Nursing Affairs, a title that enabled her to participate in the governance structures that would permit her to better understand the business and dilemmas of health care delivery and have a voice in shaping the plans for the future.

For the years that followed, she may have learned more than she felt she contributed in those meetings, but when she spoke up, she used the voice of a system executive and addressed the problem at hand, rather than the issues of the School alone. When with the president, provost, and deans, she contributed to thinking about the issues they all faced. When engaged with her faculty, she encouraged them to collaborate with others in the health system, to develop new programs and novel educational opportunities, collaborations with faculty across the campus, and coursework that brought nursing closer to the nonnurses in the campus community. Within a few years, the collaborations across the entities within the academic health center and the campus were thriving, and the faculty members were highly engaged in the work of the university.

DISCUSSION

These are just a few of the examples of nurse leaders within Duke medicine. Altogether a total of six nurses are members of the DUHS Executive Management Committee. They represent a significant proportion of the total members, and their opinions are sought as decisions are made by that group.

Why do these nurses succeed in their leadership work? As illustrated in the brief profiles of our colleagues, there are at least six common characteristics of their leadership work.

- They understand what is expected of them within their reporting structures and by those they lead.
- They focus on the good of the whole.
- They assume that their nursing background will be helpful to them making a contribution, but they do not call undue attention to nursing while doing their work.
- They engage a wide range of people in solving problems.
- They acknowledge the necessity of the team and the contributions of others.
- They work to anticipate the future and think strategically about how to be ready for the demands of the future.

These six approaches to their work enable the nurse leaders to engage in collaborations that are critical to solving the problems that are faced in the increasingly complex organizations from which we plan and deliver health care today. But approach alone is not sufficient to enacting a leadership role. In addition, each behaves in ways that we believe are characteristic of contemporary nursing leadership.

How does their behavior engender trust and assign appropriate leadership authority? Our colleagues are successful leaders, an accomplishment that develops with time, trial, and practice, but these leaders also behave in ways that have advanced their leadership success.

- They listen.
- They seek information about how they are perceived and they use the feedback.
- They prepare for meetings.
- They work hard between meetings.
- They read and collect information from their respective professional networks.
- They join others and collaborate in complex situations that are increasingly common in the delivery of health care.
- They set goals and related metrics and are able to show that results have been achieved.

Is nursing leadership unique? Although we would not describe nursing leadership as unique, it is characterized by a professional style that is particularly helpful to the leadership circle of the academic health center. Bailey et al. (2012) have described "Adaptive Leadership" as a way of behaving that is especially important in the delivery of patient care. Rooted in complexity science, Adaptive Leadership supports and enables others to face and adapt to the inevitable challenges faced in complex situations and complex organizations. Adaptive challenges are those in which the solution is unknown, and the solution requires learning and often adopting new beliefs (Bailey et al., 2012).

Virginia A. Henderson (1966), an early nurse theorist, proposed that,

> The unique function of the nurse is to assist the individual, sick or well, in the performance of those activities contributing to health or its recovery (or to a peaceful death) that the person would perform unaided given the necessary strength, will or knowledge, and to do this in such a way as to help the individual gain independence as rapidly as possible. (p. 55)

Consistent with Henderson's point of view on nursing, those who use the Adaptive Leadership framework understand their work to be assisting others so that they can address the challenges they face. We believe this to be characteristic of many nurses in leadership positions, and certainly those we have described as successful in our own environment. Furthermore, we propose that Adaptive Leadership is a promising framework for studying the work of nursing, whether in leadership at the bedside or in the board room.

INTO THE FUTURE

Leadership of thought and of action is called for today. Nurses have a key role in helping to bring about major reforms in health care. The future is bright for nursing, with increasing roles and responsibility, particularly in leading and providing direct primary and advanced care. Nursing's approach and the capacity of the nursing workforce are key solutions to the health care challenges we face today. Health care cost is growing at unsustainable rates with challenges of providing access and achieving consistent quality of care. In both developed and developing economies, there is growing recognition of the need for innovations that can lead to significant improvements to cost, quality, and access. Across the globe, many such innovative low-cost care delivery solutions are being developed that represent efficient approaches to care delivery that overcome many traditional barriers to receiving appropriate care.

Through research conducted by a partnership organization named the International Partnership for Innovative Healthcare Delivery (IPIHD), we have been able to identify common factors critical to the success of these innovative models. A major factor for success is to *"right-skill"* the workforce. The U.S. health care workforce is highly educated, and individual health care workers often do not perform at the top of their skill sets and training. This phenomenon results in workforce shortage and rising cost of care. In countries where a highly skilled labor force is absent, many innovators have relied on less-educated or skilled providers (e.g., lay workers, basic nurses, or community health educators) to deliver health care services that might otherwise be provided by more highly educated providers (e.g., advanced practice nurses or physicians). Task shifting allows the most highly trained providers to focus on more difficult cases, while trained "extenders" can help manage more routine, more prevalent health issues amenable to care of less acuity. We believe that U.S. health care can benefit from "right skilling" by enabling nurses to deliver and lead primary and community care. Many legal, economic, and regulatory hurdles constrain the opportunity to right skill in the United States. To do so, one would have to reform the regulatory and legislative environment. Of course, these barriers were squarely addressed in the first "key message" of the IOM report (2011), which called for nurses to *practice to the full extent of their education and training.* Beyond the initial legislative reforms required in the United States, we need to align the related financial incentives, including reimbursement and payment reform, to effectively implement innovations that fully utilize nurses at all levels of preparation. These reforms will best be advanced by nurses in partnership with other leaders in health care and beyond health care. Nursing leadership, of the sort we have described, can enlist the assistance of others and help to frame the case, nationally, regionally, or institutionally.

Modernizing nursing education and training to meet the emerging and complex needs will also require strong leadership as well as partnerships. Recently, Duke launched the DNP program, heavily subscribed to from across the globe, but a critically important resource in the advanced preparation of our health system executive in nursing. The review and critique of those outside of the discipline has strengthened the course of studies. The support of our system executives for nurses to return to the program has been based, in part, on a clear understanding of the value of the additional education. More recently, Duke School of Nursing has partnered with New Jersey Blue Cross/Blue Shield's Horizon Health Innovations to develop a certificate program preparing nurses for the role of population care coordinator. The need was obvious to the large insurance company, and the educational and innovation expertise at Duke led to a strong partnership to meet this need.

Most recently, Duke was awarded one of five Graduate Nurse Education (GNE) Demonstration projects. These 4-year awards from the U.S. Department of Health and Human Services Centers for Medicare & Medicaid Services are aimed at increasing the number of advanced practice nurses prepared to deliver care to the beneficiaries of Medicare. The development of the proposal was complex, and the development of a *successful* proposal was only possible through the collaboration among those who understood nursing education, with those who understood the graduate medical education (GME) model and its complex financing, and those who were attempting to bring about needed health care reforms within the health system. This award is an opportunity to collaborate for change that will benefit all, and it will be led by the nurses profiled in this chapter.

Looking ahead, we believe the role for nursing in the health care delivery system and especially for nurses to lead in the development and implementation of needed innovations is obvious. Moving forward successfully will require teams to collaborate on complex problems that belong to no one and everyone. Nurse leaders who focus on setting a vision, convening, and enabling others will lead successfully.

REFERENCES

Bailey, D., Docherty, S., Adams, J., Carthron, D., Corazzini, K., Day, J., . . . Anderson, R. (2012). Studying the clinical encounter with the Adaptive Leadership framework. *Journal of Healthcare Leadership, 4,* 1–9.

Henderson, V. (1966). *The nature of nursing: A definition and its implications for practice, research, and education* (p. 55). New York, NY: Macmillan.

Institute of Medicine. (2011). *The future of nursing: Leading change, advancing health.* Washington, DC: National Academy Press.

25

Summary and Future Directions

Greer Glazer and Joyce J. Fitzpatrick

Nurse leaders should be poised for change. Very many opportunities have been identified by the contributors to this book. One of the common themes across entries was that nurses are central to the changes occurring in health care and that they should seize the opportunities to be in charge of the redesign of the U.S. health care system. According to Smith, for example, nurses are the "beating heart" of the health care system. Those who wrote about the current health care system, whether they were referring to primary care, managed care, acute care, or home care services, all agreed that the changes would be great in the near future, partly based on health care reform initiatives, but also due to the current unsustainable high costs of our current system.

There was another strong theme that permeated the entries: that of the knowledge necessary for nurse leaders in health care delivery. To assume leadership roles in a new delivery system, nurse leaders are advised to understand policy and finance and the roles of all team members. According to several of our authors, we have very few nurses who understand policy. And, as Congressman La Tourette indicated, the first failing that nurses, and others, make in attempting to shape policy is they do not take the time to learn the process and how best to advance their cause.

Furthermore, leadership must be about the organizational goals, not one's individual goals. The individual leader must know herself or himself well enough to understand when his or her own desires and goals are taking precedence. Thus, self-knowledge is essential, including the understanding of how you are reflected in the eyes of others. A high level of self-confidence is essential for leadership, a level of confidence that is often lacking in nurses. One of the obvious conclusions was that there is a need for the profession to engage in leadership training (programs, institutes, and retreats), at all stages of nurses' development. Lifelong learning about leadership is key to success.

Other important developmental needs for nurse leaders include quantitative skills and technological expertise, including electronic and digital forms of communication. No longer can leaders be bystanders in the digital age, but rather must embrace the new modalities throughout their work. Yet the best technology in the world will not work without the right people, admonishes Dowling. Thus these skills must be combined with those of emotional intelligence, including understanding of self and others.

In summarizing key components of our authors' contributions, we thought it most instructive to identify a key quote from each of them. Each of the contributors has reflected on nurse leaders, and the key ingredients for the future development of nurse leaders. Here are their reflections or advice.

Alpert: I recommend that nursing schools develop a department of least invasive therapies and evaluations. This will legitimize the practice of these techniques and define nursing as the leader, researcher, and main practitioner of these techniques.

Blue: My heightened sensitivity to language inclusiveness is due to my nurse leader colleagues. Having worked in a physician-centric environment for most of my professional life, I was unaware of how the term "medical" may be perceived as an exclusive reference to physicians and consequently create a sense of exclusion for other health care professionals. Blue suggested the use of a more inclusive term: "health professional."

Cartwright: Successful senior administrators function within the organization vertically, as leaders and managers for their portfolio of responsibilities, and horizontally, as experienced critical thinkers and problem solvers, even when issues do not reside in areas for which they are directly responsible.

Collins: Autonomous caregivers, in any of the health care professions, have become an outdated modality. On the most successful teams, there is full appreciation of the skills of each participant and a respect for the suppression of egos that foster the success of the team as an enterprise. Nurse leaders have a unique opportunity to leverage their professional knowledge and expertise to bring health care team performance to greater levels. The focus on the patient and the advocacy that the patient feels from the nurse uniquely positions nurse leaders for this opportunity.

Cosby: Knowledge is power, and technical knowledge in today's world approaches absolute power. My mother gave me a competitive advantage as a university administrator because I was so accustomed to her success and achievements that I was better equipped to recognize the talent of women and include their recruitment as a critical aspect of developing a research organization.

Cromwell: No one becomes a great leader (or athlete) overnight. No one is born a great leader. Yes, genetic material and early childhood experiences shape people's personalities and make them more inclined to be good team-building managers, good teachers, or "ivy-tower" researchers. Leadership qualities, though, come through accumulated experience with a dose of natural selection.

Dowling: Informatics will continue to play a large part in health care, including in the role of nursing, but you can have the best technology in the world and it would not work without the right people.

There are two options when facing a problem—you can admire the problem or you can do something to solve it.

Gross: We can find more ways to capture lightning, to find leaders in unconventional ways and in nontraditional places. And, we need to believe—and experience is a good teacher—that leadership skills are not discipline specific and can be carried across the borders. Otherwise, we will have both a shortage in and a stultification of leadership.

Harris: In today's complex and increasingly culturally diverse environments, leaders must not only possess strong interpersonal/social skills but a high degree of overall emotional intelligence. Self-awareness, self-regulation, motivation, empathy, and social skills are key components of emotional intelligence that enable leaders to gauge how their actions are impacting others and modulate their behaviors as necessary.

Judge: The next phase is for nurses in other leadership roles and settings to accept the challenge of learning about, prioritizing, and attracting philanthropy. Individuals give the vast majority of the $298 billion in annual charity. Nurses touch the majority of those people every year in one way or another. Registered nurses are 1 out of every 100 people in the United States—1%. If nursing could achieve the same ratio in philanthropy, there would be $2.98 billion *every* year to transform the world's health through the power of nursing. A nurse leader must be able to communicate about what others—donors, business leaders, social influencers—value and know. A leader must be willing to venture into social circles of wealth that can sometimes be intimidating, and be able to find common ground for real conversation. To be a nurse leader in philanthropy, one must expose oneself to other values, interests, and priorities.

LaTourette: The art of effective leadership at the federal level is a little bit like going to a foreign country. Things go a lot more smoothly when you know the customs, practices, and language of the place you are visiting.

Maier: A number of people in the nursing profession truly believed that they did not become nurses to advocate for legislation, or to become involved politically. They became nurses to help people; attend to the sick, assist those in need, and to administer the care they were trained to provide. In their view, the motivation to enter the nursing profession had nothing to do with professional advocacy and the legislative process.

Mathis: I am asking for an upside-down approach to leadership in the health care industry. The only way we will address our world's health care needs is if the collective voice of nurses rules the day in organizational decision making. We must capture the character of our nurses—their vigilance, connection, humility, competence, drive, and sacrifice—and demonstrate the same leadership throughout our health care organizations. And we must embrace the visionary force guiding these characteristics in our nurses—deep, meaningful, personalized patient care.

Mazzolini: Nurses in Ohio and the issues important to them have been under the radar for too long. I understand that the culture of nursing, the training, and maybe the leadership has been to put the patient first, which is honorable. But to affect the change nurses hope and long for in Ohio, the culture must evolve.

Pate: We need to utilize technology and develop education that can be listened to/viewed at home and that has a stop and replay function. We need content that can be shared with all caregivers and that can be forwarded to a family member out of town. Patient-centered and family-centered care is far more than just education. It also has to do with how we treat patients.

Patterson: It is most impressive to me that the combination of a deep commitment to patient advocacy, a full embrace of collaborative practice models, use of a shared governance practice philosophy, and a commitment to evidence-based, data-driven systems has allowed the nursing profession to flourish.

Reistad: Associate with those leaders you wish to emulate. Do not even limit yourself to those leaders who are in your same field. The leadership skills of others in the other service industries can inspire you to greatness in "nursing" leadership.

Rosewarne: I think there has never been a better time for nurse leaders to move forward. The national and state changes in the delivery and reimbursement systems will continue, with nurses poised as well-trained, cost-effective leaders in the shortage-ridden primary care workforce. We will need nurse leaders at every point of entry in the existing health care system and will find their skills and understand a vital component in building a more patient-centered model in the health care workforce.

Smith: I believe that nurses and nursing are, and must be, the central point or organizing principle of any health care system. Nursing education and training will go well beyond the traditional subject areas to include integrated health care models, well-being and quality-of-life improvement tools, communication tools, family and community dynamics, understanding whole human lives, and outcome measurements.

van Amerongen: Nurse leaders for the next decades must be comfortable with analyzing data of all sorts to identify new opportunities and to validate what is currently being done.

Wartman: Eliminating the "guild mentality," changing restrictive policies and regulations that weaken the role of nursing, seeking to become a "transformational" as opposed to a "transactional" leader. For nurses in particular, transformational leadership is especially challenging, given the traditional hierarchies in the medical fields and academia. I would urge aspiring nurse leaders to think broadly, learn from the best and worst characteristics of leaders around them, and—always—put the patient first in decision making wherever possible.

Woerner: I still think that the servant leader concept plays into the weakness of nurses who want to be leaders, but do not want to take risks, fail forward, take chances, and simply stand up when necessary. It seems to me that the concept mistakes the leader/follower relationship, which is key to achieving a goal or vision. The challenge is to focus on the vision and be able to take some of the "cold pricklies" that are interspersed with the "warm fuzzies" when bringing about change.

Each of the authors views the kaleidoscope of leadership through a different lens; perhaps the particles are the same but the image is one shaped of their own experience, not just with nurse leaders but also from their experiences with health care and leaders from other disciplines.

The preceding quotes can be woven together to form a rich fabric of leadership lessons for aspiring nurse leaders. At a minimum these reflections from distinguished colleagues will provide points of discussion in the many forums developed to prepare more nurse leaders.

Index